FORGED IN FITNESS
How I Found Healing, Strength, and Purpose — so can you. Includes practical fitness & nutrition guidelines
Waldimir Robert Baskovich

Copyright © 2025 by Waldimir Robert Baskovich
All rights reserved. No part of this publication may be reproduced, stored in a retrieval system, or transmitted in any form or by any means—electronic, mechanical, photocopying, recording, or otherwise—without the prior written permission of the publisher, except in the case of brief quotations used in critical articles or reviews.

Published by Baskovich Publishing
Printed in the United States of America

ISBN 979-8-218-76465-4 (Paperback)
ISBN 979-8-218-76466-1 (E-book)

All applicable copyright laws enforced.

Scripture quotations are primarily taken from the King James Version (KJV). Other translations used include the New International Version (NIV), New English Translation (NET), and the World English Bible (WEB), unless otherwise noted.

Updated January 2026

Dedication

This book is a tribute to my father, Waldimir Baskovich—a true legacy of strength who provided a solid foundation, instilled a never-quit attitude, and showed through his life what perseverance and discipline truly mean.

He grew up in poverty in St. Louis, MO, the eldest of four siblings. Sacrifice wasn't a concept he learned later in life—it was his starting point. At just eleven years old, while collecting coal near the rumbling tracks to help heat his family's home, he lost his left leg in a tragic accident. That moment could have defined him as broken. For many, it would have. But not him.

Instead of being defeated, he chose to rise. That loss became the foundation of his determination. He didn't just overcome it, he used it to build something greater: strength of character, unwavering focus, and the kind of determination that inspires generations.

He adapted, defied limits, and refused to let circumstances dictate his fate. A leather strap on his bike pedal symbolized his mindset: find a way, no excuses. Through relentless effort, he became a three-time AAU gold medalist on the flying rings in the 1940s—the first amputee in America to achieve this distinction—and later a two-time U.S. amputee golf champion.

His success wasn't solely athletic; it was also spiritual. He built businesses, supported his family, and upheld values that couldn't be taught in school—only earned through grit. He rarely said, "I love you," but he demonstrated it through his actions, integrity, humility, consistency, and an unshakable belief that nothing is impossible.

"Today, I honor him for all he endured and became, and for the strength he passed on to our family. His legacy lives on in every challenge I face with resolve and in every step I take without surrender."

I also I want to thank my mother, for whose prayers sustained me throughout my youth.

Contents

Disclaimer	IX
Introduction	X
1. MY CHAOTIC YOUTH	1
Early Lessons in Fear – My Near Drowning	
Made Powerless — Bullied and Adrift	
The Illusion of Freedom — Counterculture and Escape	
Dazed & Confused with Social Anxiety	
2. WHEN FITNESS BECAME SACRED	14
That's where it began.	
Fitness is Deeply Personal	
Never Be Easy On Yourself	
Fitness Became More Than a Routine, It Became Sacred	
Life Is Fleeting	
Quotes That Carved My Path	
3. FITNESS GUIDELINES	29
Resistance Training	
Circuit Training and HIIT: Efficient & Effective	
Weightlifting & Cardio: Best Sequence for Fat Burn	
Exercises for Runners	
My Fitness Principles	
Mistakes Made at the Gym	
Goal Met, Now What?	
4. EFFECTIVE WORKOUT PLANS	41
Choose Your Approach	
Finding What Works for You	

    Workout Styles to Explore
    A Basic Well-Rounded Weekly Weightlifting Guide

5. IMPORTANCE OF RESISTANCE TRAINING   51
    Proper Muscle Contraction – Key to Results
    Key Concepts of TUT – Time Under Tension
    Lactate Threshold
    NEGATIVE & ISOMETRIC TRAINING
    Mind-Muscle Connection
    Make Each Rep Count
    The Myth Of Muscle Confusion

6. STRENGTH TRAINING FOR FAT LOSS MATTERS   73
    The Problem With Cardio-Only Weight Loss
    Why Strength Training Wins
    The Foundation: Compound Movements
    Why The Scale Goes Up Before It Goes Down
    Roadblocks to Weight Loss

7. HIGHLY EFFECTIVE EXERCISE METHODOLOGIES   85
    The Best Go-To's
    Explosive Power & Reactive Training
    Interval & Circuit Training
    Exercising With A Bad Back

8. BREATH CONTROL = BETTER PERFORMANCE   92
    For Resistance & High-Intensity Exercises
    Running, or Walking

9. WALKING & CHI RUNNING   96
    Walk For Fat Loss and Function
    Interval Walking = Next Level
    Core Concepts of Chi Running

10. AB EXERCISES. BELLY FAT. SWEAT IT OFF?   100
    Abdominal Exercises
    Abdominal Obesity
    The Truth About Belly Fat Loss
    Visceral Fat

More Sweat, Burn More Fat?

11. STRONG MOTHERS — 111
    Will Women Get Bulky?
    Muscle Tone Vs. Bulk

12. SENIOR EXERCISES — 120
    Getting Started Safely
    Exercise Classes & Sports for Those New to Fitness
    Longevity —Thriving: Quality of Life

13. BEHAVIORAL STRATEGIES — 130
    The Psychology Behind Sustainable Change
    Rewire Your Brain With Self-Talk & Discipline

14. NUTRITION — Eat Like Your Life Depends on it — 136
    Calories In vs. Out Isn't the Whole Picture
    Macronutrients

15. EFFECTIVE DIETS AND GUIDELINES — 146
    Why Do Some Diet Books Fail, While Others Work?
    Grace-Based Eating Principles
    Nutrition For Performance
    Creatine & BCAAs
    GOOD, NOT SO GOOD
    Basic Foods You Can Eat Often
    Foods You Can Eat in Moderation

    Foods to Never Eat (or Avoid as Much as Possible)
    Ultra-Processed Foods
    Harmful Effects of Sugar
    CARBS, FAT, FIBER
    Alkaline Water & Acidic Foods
    Hydration Check: Urine Color & What It Means

16. PROTEIN: YOUR TOP PRIORITY — 181
    Thermogenetic Effect of Protein & Weight Management
    Buying Fish: Fresh Or Frozen?
    10 Signs You're Not Eating Enough Protein

17. MEAL REPLACEMENTS 193
    Animal Protein Sources
    Plant-Based Proteins
    Carbohydrate Sources
    Fat Sources
    Food Hacks
    Protein Hacks
    Nutritious Power Bowls & Snacks

18. SAFE & SUSTAINABLE FAT LOSS 208
    Fat Loss Facts & Spot Reduction Myths
    Metabolic Shift After Weight Loss

DAILY REMINDER CHART 216

A TRAINER GUIDED BY GOD'S HEART 218

EPILOGUE 219
    The Battle That Challenged Everything

ABOUT THE AUTHOR 222

Disclaimer

Disclaimer & Release of Liability

The information in this book is intended for general guidance and educational purposes only. It is not a substitute for professional medical advice, diagnosis, or treatment. Always consult your physician or a qualified healthcare provider before starting any exercise, nutrition, or wellness program—especially if you have pre-existing health conditions, injuries, or medical concerns.

The author, publisher, and contributors are not licensed medical professionals and accept no liability for injuries, health complications, or damages resulting from the use or misuse of the content presented in this book. By participating in any exercises, training routines, or nutritional suggestions, you accept full responsibility for your own health and safety.

Physical activity carries inherent risks, including but not limited to injury, strain, or the aggravation of existing conditions. By using this book, you acknowledge and voluntarily accept these risks, releasing the author, publisher, affiliates, and associated parties from all liability, claims, or causes of action.

Introduction

This is not just a book. It is an invitation to elevate yourself—not at some distant point in a perfect future, but right here, in the middle of confusion, setbacks, and quiet struggles. It is a call to discover strength where most people are taught to believe none exists.

I understand what it feels like to fall. To lose direction. To wake up and wonder how you ended up so far from who you thought you might become. I've lived through fear, isolation, and long stretches of disconnection—both from others and from myself. I know what it means to drift without purpose and to sense, deep down, that the path you're on leads nowhere good.

For me, the turning point did not arrive as clarity or inspiration. It arrived as movement. Fitness—specifically weight training and martial arts—began as a way to quiet the noise in my head. Over time, it became something far more important. Through disciplined movement, I rebuilt more than my body. I rebuilt direction, resilience, and a sense of internal order that the world had slowly stripped away. Strength became more than physical; it became a way to engage with life instead of hiding from it.

This book is built on that process. Not theory. Not trends. Not motivational fluff. What you'll find here comes from lived experience and practical application—principles that helped me move from survival to stability, and from instability to purpose. The focus is not perfection. It is progress earned through effort, consistency, and honest self-assessment.

Pain and progress often travel together. Fear does not disappear when you grow stronger—you learn to move through it. Setbacks are inevitable; they are not the measure of a person. The response is. Real transformation is not a single moment of insight. It is the accumulation of imperfect, courageous steps taken in the right direction.

If you are looking for a shortcut, this book is not for you. If you are willing to engage in the work—physical, mental, and personal—this book offers a framework to help you rebuild strength, clarity, and confidence from the inside out.

The pages that follow are not an excuse, a confession, or a dramatization of the past. They are context. They explain the ground I started from, the patterns I had to confront, and why lasting change required more than motivation alone. Everything that came after—the damage and the rebuilding—rests on that foundation.

If you've ever felt stuck, lost, or invisible in your struggle, understand this: you are not alone—and your story is not finished.

Chapter 1
MY CHAOTIC YOUTH

I never set out to become who I am today. My growth wasn't fueled by ambition, discipline, or a specific goal. Rather, it was molded by a sequence of experiences that initially generated fear, then helplessness, and eventually revealed how straightforward it can be to conquer both.

At the time, none of these experiences seemed significant. They were not milestones or obvious turning points. No single moment felt decisive. They were simply events that left marks—subtle at first, then cumulative.

What mattered was not their severity, but their repetition. Each encounter reinforced the same lesson: control can be taken away quickly, sometimes without warning and often without explanation. When this happens often enough, you stop searching for meaning and start searching for relief. Fear becomes familiar. Helplessness becomes routine. Escape begins to feel less like a choice and more like a strategy.

I did not understand this process while it was happening. I only felt its effects. My responses to stress, how I treated my own body, and how I defined strength were all quietly shaped during this period. Long before I ever thought about discipline, recovery, or rebuilding, I was learning the opposite lessons—how to brace, how to withdraw, how to numb.

This chapter is not a highlight reel, nor is it an attempt to dramatize the past. It exists because these early experiences formed the mental framework I carried forward. They explain the ground I started on, the patterns I developed, and why later change required more than motivation alone.

What follows is not an excuse or a confession. It is context. Everything that came after—the damage and the rebuilding—rests on this foundation.

Early Lessons in Fear – My Near Drowning

At the tender age of eight, my world often centered around the boundaries of our backyard fishpond. That small corner of our property became the core of my universe. It wasn't large—just a simple rectangle roughly three feet deep, four feet wide, and ten feet long. To an adult, it was nothing more than a modest stone pond in our backyard, a simple water feature with a solid ring of rocks that kept the water contained. It held a lively group of goldfish that flashed orange and white beneath the surface, weaving between shadows, stones, and drifting leaves.

But to me, that pond was an entire world. It was an enchanted realm where my imagination could breathe and grow. In my mind, it constantly changed: sometimes it was an ocean with hidden depths; other times, a fortress with invisible walls; occasionally, it became a secret kingdom where only I knew the rules. It was my place, my territory, the one spot where the rest of life faded into the background.

I memorized every detail of it—the shape of the stones around its edges, the subtle patterns the sunlight created as it filtered through tree branches, the quiet ripples that spread when the wind touched the water. I would circle this pond endlessly on my cherished Schwinn. The metallic rattle of the handlebars, the hum of the tires, the crackle of twigs and dried leaves beneath my feet all blended into a familiar rhythm that defined my childhood. Those sounds, combined with the buzzing insects and birds overhead, formed a soundtrack I felt belonged only to me.

Over time, my daily rides became more than just routine. They felt like a silent agreement between me and the Earth beneath me, as if the ground recognized me as its rightful traveler. The stones around the pond marked the boundary of my kingdom, and every lap I rode felt ceremonial. I would pause at the same spot and rest my foot on the largest stone, feeling its coolness through the sole of my sneaker. That simple act felt grounding and steady. It made me confident. It made me feel like I belonged there.

I confidently took charge of that space—until suddenly, the earth decided it didn't want to cooperate anymore.

I rode along the edge with the same certainty I had felt hundreds of times before. But without warning, the balance I trusted betrayed me. My foot slipped off the stone it had always rested on. In an instant, the world tilted sharply. Gravity took over, pulling me down with a speed and force that stunned me. The pond welcomed me without hesitation. The water opened itself and swallowed me whole.

The cold shock hit me immediately. I plunged to the bottom faster than my mind could catch up. Before I could orient myself, my Schwinn followed me into the water and crashed down across my small body, pressing me into the slim at the bottom. The weight of it pinned me entirely. The pond floor felt slimy and alien, and the water's darkness distorted everything.

The stones that surrounded the pond—my stones—now formed a jagged wall above me. The surface of the water seemed impossibly far away. What had once been a place of play now felt like a sealed chamber.

My instincts told me to lift the bike upward, sliding it along the wall of the pond until it broke through the top. I pressed the tires against the pond wall and slowly slid them up, inch by inch, forcing the bike to rise with me.

But it wasn't enough. Just as the tires neared the top, they hit the overhanging stones that framed the pond's edge. Those stones, which always looked decorative and harmless from above, now acted like a ledge that blocked any upward movement. The bike was jammed under the lip of the rock. I could slide it no more farther. No matter how hard I pushed, the tires stopped cold against that barrier.

That was the moment the truth hit me: I might not get out.

The panic that swept through me was pure, electric fear. My lungs burned. My heart pounded in my chest. For the first time in my short life, I understood what it meant to be completely trapped.

And then it happened.

The fear vanished—completely and instantly. A deep calm flooded through me, warm and quiet, as if someone had wrapped a blanket of stillness around my heart. My breathing slowed. My thoughts cleared. Instead of frantic terror, I experienced a peace I couldn't explain.

I became aware of something else—a presence, not seen but unmistakably felt. It was as if a gentle force stepped in, quieting everything inside me. Time no longer flowed. The water around me stopped feeling cold. The panic dissolved into serenity.

In that brief moment of stillness, my body adjusted. The bike, which had halted a moment before, tilted slightly to the right, creating a gap. I slid sideways and then rose.

My head broke through the surface, and the air slammed into my lungs—sharp, sweet, overwhelming. I gasped again and again, grabbing the stones at the edge and pulling myself out of the pond. I stood on the solid ground, trembling, soaked, but alive.

As the water dripped from my clothes, I felt something inside me settle into place. I had brushed up against something far bigger than fear or childhood imagination. Whatever steadied me beneath the surface wasn't instinct or luck. It felt guided.

Even at eight years old, I understood that I had been helped. The peace I felt underwater wasn't shock or numbness—it was something pure, protective, and entirely beyond explanation. I believed—without hesitation—that an angel, or something very close to one, had intervened.

That moment became a defining point in my life. The serenity I felt at the bottom of that pond remains one of my clearest memories. Even now, when I think back on it, I can still sense a trace of that stillness, that warmth, that presence.

It wasn't the danger that stayed with me. It was the overwhelming peace.

It was the first time I ever sensed something Heavenly, something protective, something undeniably real.

Made Powerless — Bullied and Adrift

Growing up, I often felt like I was just drifting — present, but not truly part of things. I showed up, I walked the halls, I sat in classrooms, but it always felt like I was floating a few inches outside my own life. I wasn't absent, but I wasn't fully there either. I felt like someone watching life through a pane of glass, close enough to see everything but somehow blocked from touching it. I wasn't the smartest kid in class, not the fastest on the field, and definitely not the loudest in the room. I lived in that quiet, middle ground where you exist, but no one really notices you're there. I wasn't disliked; I just wasn't seen. I stayed somewhere in the background, unsure, observing more than participating, quietly searching for a place to belong.

Other kids seemed to navigate life easily. They laughed loudly in crowded hallways, leaning shoulder-to-shoulder in groups that felt like tribes. They belonged without needing to earn it. Their confidence appeared natural, as if they were born with it. They had their cliques, inside jokes, quick laughter, and a natural rhythm that made everything seem simple. I wanted to understand that world, to know what it felt like to walk into a room and feel welcomed, wanted, and included. But every time I got close, something inside me froze. It wasn't fear of them — it was fear of not fitting in, fear of being exposed as someone out of place.

I'd see the "in" crowd walking toward me, and instinctively I'd turn down another hallway or pretend I needed something from my locker. It wasn't cowardice. It was a form of self-defense, a quiet truth I knew even then: I didn't belong in their orbit. Their world felt unreachable, like a radio station I could hear but never quite tune into. Close enough to tease me, but just far enough to remain impossible.

I talked to people, sure, but never the ones with that effortless confidence. My conversations were surface-level — polite nods, quick comments, small talk that kept everything safe and controlled. Deep down, I was waiting for something I couldn't define — a purpose, a spark, a direction that would pull me out of that quiet fog I lived in. I wanted to matter. I wanted to find something that made sense of me. I didn't want to stay invisible forever. I just didn't know how to rise — not yet.

There were days I felt invisible, and other days when I wished I truly was. I still remember the cold slam of a locker door against my back — the echo that vibrated through my spine, the sting, the metallic smell that lingered in the air afterward. Older boys — the jocks, the ones everyone treated like they were untouchable — cornered/**bullied** me more than once. They didn't need to hit me. Their tone alone made it clear I had no choice. They demanded my lunch tickets, and even though it didn't happen often, maybe just a handful of times, the fear carved itself deep into me. My hands trembled every time I handed those tickets over, not because of the loss, but because of the helplessness.

After that, I learned how to vanish. I studied the hallways like a soldier studies enemy moves — scanning for danger, memorizing patterns, finding the safest paths. I took routes where no one walked. I avoided eye contact. My world shrank into safe zones: the quiet corner of the library where the sunlight fell just right; the far end of the lunchroom where kids kept to themselves; the spaces where no one cared enough to look. Each day became a mission: stay small, stay unseen, survive.

But suppression always has a cost. Fear doesn't just disappear; it condenses, sinks deeper, and hardens. Beneath the surface, that fear turns into shame, which eventually sharpens into anger — not the loud kind that explodes outward, but the quiet, simmering type that twists inside you. It becomes a pressure you avoid talking about, a knot you can't untie, a shadow you carry like an extra limb.

That buried ember stayed hidden for years, but it never went out. And then, when I was about fourteen, something inside me snapped loose.

I don't know what triggered it. Maybe it was exhaustion from carrying that quiet resentment for so long. Maybe it was the buildup of too many days spent swallowing my emotions. Maybe I just wanted, for one reckless moment, to understand what power felt like — real power, the kind I saw in the boys who never had to look over their shoulders. Whatever the reason, I crossed a line. I once swore I never would.

I became what I hated.

I pushed a younger kid hard — harder than I intended and more than he deserved. The crash of him hitting the ground felt unusually loud, echoing in the startling silence that followed, which seemed too empty and still. I gazed down at him, and a voice erupted from me that didn't sound like my own — sharp, tense, driven by an uncalled-for rage. My hands moved involuntarily, mechanical and foreign, as if they weren't mine. For a brief moment, a wave of dominance surged through me — electric, shocking, almost addictive.

And then it vanished.

What replaced it wasn't satisfaction or triumph. It was emptiness. A hollow drop in my stomach. A disgust that hit harder than any punch. I'd crossed into a territory I didn't want to be in. I had become the thing that once terrified me.

That moment haunted me—not just because of what I'd done, but because of what it revealed. Pain, if ignored long enough, can turn into something unrecognizable. I had carried that weight on my chest for years, and in a single moment, I put that same burden on someone else. That realization cut deep.

How had my pain so easily turned into cruelty?
How had my soul bent so quickly under pressure?
Why was it so effortless to become the very thing I despised?

Those questions didn't fade. They lingered long after the guilt set in. That moment might have seemed small or forgettable to anyone watching, but to me, it was monumental. It taught me something stark: when weakness isn't confronted, it mutates. It becomes dangerous. Not just to you — but to anyone you touch.

By the end of junior high, I'd only been in a few fights — if you could even call them fights. A few punches thrown here and there, moments of chaos rather than skill. Nothing that shapes a boy into a man. But those moments did teach me something important: becoming a man isn't about the number of fights you survive or the bruises you collect. It's about the battles you fight inside yourself — the ones no one sees.

Manhood isn't built through violence.
It's built through restraint.

By having the courage to remain calm when everything inside is urging to burst, and learning to communicate instead of lash out, to seek understanding rather than control, true strength isn't about intimidation—it's about self-restraint. It's the awareness that you could cause harm but opting not to.

Manhood isn't formed in fists.
It's formed in fire — the kind that burns inside until you learn how to control it.
That was the beginning of mine.

> *Like Daniel in the lion's den, a godly man faces trials with courage and unwavering faith, knowing that each challenge is a chance to grow stronger.*

The Illusion of Freedom — Counterculture and Escape

My later teenage years felt like a blur — chaotic, unstable, and spinning toward an uncertain future. The world around me was changing, and I was changing with it, whether I wanted to or not. Everything that once felt solid seemed to loosen its hold. The 1960s **hippie counterculture** was sweeping through the country, and even if you didn't actively participate, its influence touched everyone. The music, attitudes, and spirit of rebellion infiltrated our daily lives. High school, which ideally would have been a clear, steady route to adulthood, instead turned into a battleground—fighting over identity, temptation, and illusions rather than just grades or popularity.

The noise was constant. Radios blared garage bands in every neighborhood. Kids gathered on porches, in cars, and behind schools, talking loudly about freedom, questioning rules, and pushing boundaries none of us truly understood. Conversations focused on rebellion, living without restraint, doing what felt good, and tearing down anything that resembled structure. Everyone wanted to break free from something, even if most of us couldn't clearly explain what that "something" was. What seemed like freedom at first was intoxicating, but beneath it was confusion — a current pulling us further away from ourselves than we realized.

The movement's vibrant exterior — the music, the slogans, the talk of liberation — concealed something darker underneath. There was a slow erosion hidden beneath all that color and noise, a quiet hollowing out. It whispered to us that we were becoming enlightened, awakened, liberated. But in reality, what seemed like discovery was actually disassembly. Piece by piece, I was taking myself apart and calling it growth.

I drifted through those years like a ship without a compass, sails full but lacking direction. I kept searching for meaning or something to fill the hollow silence I carried inside. I didn't know what I was looking for — purpose, belonging, confidence, or identity — it all blurred together. Marijuana became my constant companion. Not for excitement, but for escape. It wrapped me in a gentle fog that softened everything. Problems blurred. Pain dulled. Questions quieted. For a short time, it made life feel easier. But underneath that false calm, the emptiness deepened.

Weekends became my safe haven, a little escape just for me. I wasn't partying to celebrate anything special, but rather using the smoke as a way to hide — from the pain of my failures, from the weight of unmet expectations, and from the quiet heaviness that felt so overwhelming at times. Getting high wasn't rebellion for me. It was avoidance. It let me drift without having to face myself. I told myself that meant freedom, that I was breaking away from the grip of society, that I was "thinking differently." But that was a lie. I wasn't running toward anything new. I was running away — fast, blind, and without considering where it led.

The so-called hippie lifestyle wrapped itself around me like a soft lie. It promised freedom, peace, authenticity—a life without rules or judgment. None of it held up. Every high hollowed me out a little more. The quiet afterward was heavier than the noise. The harder I chased feeling alive, the more I disappeared. What looked like freedom from the outside was really a slow, silent slide into nothing. On top of that, I was buried in weekend drinking binges, numbing whatever was left.

Promiscuity became another mask. It wasn't about desire or connection, and it wasn't anything romantic. It was about control, or at least pretending to have it. We called it "free love," but mostly it was insecurity wearing the costume of confidence. We were trying to feel significant through motion, hoping contact would fill the void inside. It didn't. Beneath the peace signs and slogans, there was no awakening — only escape, another layer of noise to drown out the silence.

We told ourselves we were enlightened. The truth was simpler: we were lost. Too young to understand the gravity of our choices, too restless to slow down, too stubborn to admit we were destroying ourselves. We confused chaos with purpose, rebellion with strength. We thought if we blurred every line long enough, answers would emerge from the haze. But the only thing that sharpened was the emptiness inside us.

The warning signs hit hard and fast. I saw them written on faces I once admired. Two former honor students — kids who had once been sharp, driven, full of potential — disappeared into the fog of LSD. When I looked into their eyes, I saw nothing looking back. The spark, the intelligence that once shone through them had vanished. No longer rebels or visionaries, they were now casualties—ghosts trapped in a nightmare they couldn't even recognize as such.

That image still haunts me. Even now, decades later, I can feel the chill from that realization. That should have been enough to wake me up — to shock me back into clarity. But it didn't. I kept going anyway, too numb to care, too stubborn to admit to myself that I was walking the same path they were.

The truth is, no one forced me into any of it. The crowd I hung out with was my choice. I sought them out. I walked into those basements and dimly lit rooms alone. I stayed through the smoke-filled nights, listening to the same conversations circling the same dead ends. I bought drugs from anyone who had them—friends, acquaintances, strangers. It didn't matter. I didn't ask questions because I didn't want to hear the answers. I just wanted the next high, the next distraction, the next way to quiet the ache. Looking back, I see clearly that I was dancing with death each time. And the fact that I survived isn't luck — it's grace.

And if you find yourself caught in that same current — or watching someone you love drift toward it — remember this: it doesn't have to end there. You can turn around. You can walk away. You can break the pattern before it breaks you. It won't be easy. It might be the hardest step you ever take. But it's the one that leads to life, an awakening.

Find something that challenges you — something that builds instead of destroys. A sport, a discipline, or a pursuit that requires structure and focus. Gyms became that space for me — not for vanity or ego, but for order. For direction. For a sense of progress. The right environment and the right people can be a turning point. Surround yourself with those who lift you higher, not those who pull you down.

For me, martial arts became the forge. A good dojo is sacred ground — not because of the mats or the equipment, but because of what the discipline asks of you. Under a strong teacher, the chaos inside you gradually finds direction. You learn to master not the people around you, but the storm within you. The rituals, the repetition, the respect — they create structure in a mind that once felt unstructured. Each class chips away at weakness and replaces it with resolve. The lessons seep into every corner of your life. Stand tall. Stay focused. Act with honor. Control the fire instead of letting it burn you.

Gradually, the fog started to lift. It wasn't a single moment of clarity, but a buildup of small ones. My mother's prayers. The memory of those empty, LSD-drained eyes. The quiet voice inside me that refused to die, no matter how hard I tried to drown it out. Each moment pushed me forward.

Step by step, I started to move again. I didn't notice at first, but the discipline my father lived by — the drive, the persistence, the unwillingness to quit — began to come alive in me. Small actions led to bigger ones. A short run became part of my routine. A workout became a commitment. A goal turned into a path.

Pain shifted from something I avoided to something I learned to rely on. Instead of fleeing from it, I started to use it — as fuel, as guidance, as a reminder that I was still capable of change. The body I had neglected for so long slowly became the instrument of my renewal. Those early steps didn't resolve everything, but they marked the start of a turning point — the moment when drifting turned into direction. The boy who once sought numbness was learning how to feel. And on that foundation, strength, purpose, and faith gradually began to take shape.

Dazed & Confused with Social Anxiety

My mind was at war with itself — caught in a relentless storm of confusion and fear I couldn't quiet. I was about twenty, attending a grand family wedding in Indiana. Nearly five hundred guests filled the banquet hall. Laughter, perfume, and clinking glasses drifted through the room like smoke curling through beams of warm light. The chatter rose into a single, swirling hum — familiar to everyone else but strangely foreign to me. I stood in the middle of it all, frozen and detached, as if watching life unfold through frosted glass.

From the moment I arrived, something inside me shifted. At first, it was subtle — a faint static in the back of my mind — but it grew quickly, multiplying, thickening, and tightening. The fog rolled in softly but heavily, dulling every color and muffling every sound until the entire room felt both too close and unreachable all at once. Every smile appeared forced. Every cheer sounded hollow. Every toast seemed rehearsed. Even the tiny bride and groom figures on top of the cake looked more alive than the people celebrating around me.

The chandelier's golden light spilled across the hall, but instead of warmth, I felt the cold efficiency of distance — like I was floating outside myself. My hands flexed, then curled into fists without my consent. My chest tightened. The edges of the room distorted. I could see everything, yet nothing felt real.

Was this my life… or just a distorted reflection of it?

The feeling wasn't new. I had experienced this strange detachment for years — lurking in crowded hallways, busy streets, even simple family gatherings. Small groups were tolerable, sometimes even comforting. But large ones made me feel unmoored, like gravity had loosened and I might drift away if I wasn't careful. My heart would race. My skin would turn cold. Sounds blended together until they felt like waves crashing inside my head. I'd be surrounded by people, yet feel completely alone.

In those moments, I had a ritual — a strange, personal survival tactic. I would find a mirror. Any mirror. A bathroom, a hallway, or even a window with enough reflection. If I could stare into my own eyes long enough, I could ground myself. *You are here. You are real.* Those words had saved me countless times.

But at that wedding, they slipped through my fingers.

The pressure in my chest became unbearable, swelling like a balloon stretched to its limit. Laughter in the room no longer sounded joyful — it sounded sharp, intrusive, like a wall of noise closing in on me. The air grew thin, too cold and too tight to breathe. I felt trapped in a world that suddenly felt foreign.

I needed to get out. Now.

Without thinking or planning, I turned and pushed through the crowd. The music pounded in my chest with heavy, uneven beats. The scent of cologne, perfume, and champagne filled my nose like a chemical haze. I moved faster, weaving between tables, brushing against coats and dresses, ignoring the surprised faces and questions. The large doors at the end of the hall seemed like a gateway from a dream I was hesitant to leave.

I burst through them and stumbled into the night.

Cold air hit me in the face — crisp, clean, almost sharp. My lungs expanded, but the panic didn't quiet down. In fact, the cold made it worse. My breathing became short, uneven bursts, as if my body had forgotten how to breathe. The parking lot stretched out in long shadows, and for a moment I lost sense of where I was or which way led to safety. My mind demanded control, something familiar, any sign of grounding.

Somehow, through the fog of fear, my body moved on instinct. I don't even remember making the decision — one moment I was outside the hall, and the next I was in my car, hands trembling on the wheel. Everything around me looked warped, like I was driving through a tunnel with no clear sense of distance or time. Streetlights stretched into streaks. The road felt unfamiliar, even though I'd driven it earlier that day. My mind couldn't hold a straight thought, but my hands kept steering, turning onto streets I barely recognized. I followed a path my memory couldn't consciously trace, guided more by instinct than awareness. I don't know how long it took to reach the hotel. It could've been minutes or an hour — the world felt distorted, stretched thin, unreal. All I knew was that somehow, despite the panic crushing my chest, the car carried me back.

When I finally got to the room, the door shut behind me like a vault sealing shut. I collapsed on the bed, my chest rising and falling unevenly as the adrenaline drained from my body. When it left, it took everything with it—strength, clarity, even the ability to think clearly. Sleep came in fragments, shallow and restless. I floated in and out, caught in a strange space between waking and falling asleep, never quite reaching true rest.

Peace did not follow.

Not long after, as the episodes grew stronger and harder to hide, my parents took me to a psychiatrist. I was prescribed medication meant to quiet the anxiety and steady the storm. But for me, it only deepened the fog. I already felt unreal — and the pills pushed me further away from myself. My thoughts dulled. My emotions blurred. The sense of disconnection became thicker and more suffocating.

I knew I couldn't surrender my mind so easily.

I made a choice — not out of rebellion, but out of necessity. I refused the medication and decided to fight on my own terms. I don't say that as advice. There were later seasons when medication helped me, when it was right and necessary. But at that age, in that moment, refusing it was my first declaration of war against the darkness. It was the first time I said, "I'm not letting fear define me."

Still, the battle continued. The fear of crowds clung to me like a persistent shadow, silent but always nearby. It followed me through my early adulthood, shaping my decisions, shrinking my world, and controlling where I went and how I lived. To others, I appeared normal. To me, the anxiety was everywhere — a constant hum beneath the surface. Sometimes I wondered if it ran in my blood, a generational wound quietly passed down through time.

I have never fully understood it. Maybe I never will. Invisible wounds rarely show themselves openly; yet, they leave scars — subtle, deep, and lasting. Even after the worst episodes had faded, their echoes lingered for some time. Small incidents brought back distant whispers of fear. A crowded room, a sudden noise, sensory overload — not enough to overpower me anymore, but enough to remind me of where I've come from.

I knew I needed something—a foundation, a focus, a discipline to hold onto when the world felt unreal. That anchor became fitness. Initially, it was about survival. Later, it shifted to building structure, leading to transformation. The kicks, repetitions, sweat, and training rhythm did more than develop skill and muscle; they created stability. Discipline brought order amid chaos. The physical aspect steadied the mental.

Over time, training became something sacred. It turned into meditation in motion — every set and rep a battle cry against fear. Each workout was a deliberate return to presence, a reminder that I was here, alive, real. I gradually learned that **true strength isn't about controlling everything — it's about showing up fully, mentally and physically, in the moment you're in.**

Scripture and truth started carving clarity where confusion once reigned. Faith gave me words for battles I'd never previously been able to label. I stopped chasing illusions and began building an inner fortress — steady, grounded, authentic.

The anxiety didn't vanish overnight. But it no longer controlled me. It still appeared sometimes, but **I had built something stronger: discipline, faith, and a solid foundation that could withstand the storm.**

And in that shift — in that hard-earned freedom — I learned something: Strength isn't the absence of fear.
Strength is the ability to move forward despite it.

Chapter 2
WHEN FITNESS BECAME SACRED

Even in a warm, loving home, a child can sometimes feel lost. My parents were truly wonderful—my mother gentle and full of love, my father steady and caring in his quiet, reassuring way. I was supported and safe. Yet even with all of that, I often found myself drifting. Not because of them, but because each of us must eventually walk a path of our own.

Gradually, I began to notice a change in me—at first, barely perceptible. My mother's prayers, subtle yet unwavering, felt like seeds quietly taking root in my heart. At the same time, I felt a growing desire to escape—not simply from the noise around me, but from the confusion within. The people, the choices, the paths being offered all felt hollow. None of it seemed to lead anywhere meaningful.

It was during this time that I began to see my father's example in a new light.

When I was a boy—elementary school age—he had me get up early for a few years and train. Nothing elaborate. About twenty minutes. Basic calisthenics. A little running around the house, sometimes up and down the block. I did it because he asked me to. That was simply a way of life.

Some mornings I loved it. Other mornings I hated it. Eventually, I complained enough that he had me stop. He didn't argue or force the issue. He simply let it go.

I could no longer pretend that everything inside me was fine. The noise and empty promises felt untrustworthy and chaotic. My spirit was fragile, easily pulled off course. I longed for something solid—something structured, something real. **In my late teens, I stepped back and began searching: for truth, for peace, for people who trained their bodies, sharpened their minds, and lived with purpose.**

That's where it began.

Fitness was never about appearance. It became a way of discovering myself—one rep, one workout, one disciplined day at a time. **This marked a turning point. I stopped drifting and began forging my own path.** What followed didn't just transform my body; it reshaped my entire life.

My sister recognized that I was struggling and introduced me to her friend, Sensei John B., a martial arts instructor. That introduction led me to the dojo, where I was exposed to discipline, respect, and self-control. Around the same time, I began basic weightlifting—simple, consistent, dependable. Together, these practices became grounding forces for a restless mind that needed direction.

At first, fitness was an escape—a way to break free from destructive habits and negative influences. I was often overwhelmed by the weight of my own decisions. But with each kick, each repetition, and every drop of sweat, something deeper began to take shape. I wasn't just gaining strength; I was reconnecting with my sense of self-worth. Martial arts and weightlifting gave me focus, structure, and a reason to stay present. They also restored hope.

The storm didn't pass overnight, but it quieted enough for me to hear what had been buried beneath the noise. Slowly, I began to recognize who I truly was.

Here's a reminder worth holding onto: when your thoughts become tangled and overwhelming, resist the urge to silence them. Instead, listen with patience—like an orchestra tuning before the music begins. Clarity often follows chaos. Your mind doesn't need to be perfect; it needs time, faith, and compassion. Think of yourself as the conductor, learning to guide your thoughts and shape your own harmony.

> This mindset helped me focus on building a real connection rather than trying to control everything. It kept me connected to what's real. If you're reading this, I hope these words remind you of your inner strength. We're all in this storm together, and remember, you're never alone.

Fitness is Deeply Personal

What works for one person may not work for another. Age, experience, physical limitations, and individual goals all play a crucial role in shaping what your ideal training approach looks like. That's why I strongly recommend working with a qualified coach or personal trainer—someone who can tailor a program to your specific needs and guide you safely and effectively.

Covering every method, movement, and variation in one book would take volumes—and even then, it couldn't match the evolving science and art of training. This isn't an academic thesis but a practical, proven guide based on science, experience, and results from athletes, clients, and my five decades in fitness. I don't claim to know everything, but I've spent a lifetime learning, testing, and refining what I believe works.

This section offers a framework of principles and sample structures you can build on, regardless of your starting point. I've kept it simple because progress comes from consistency, proper guidance, and smart effort—not complexity. When researching, rely on reputable, science-based sources—not trends or social media hype. Think of this as a compass, not a detailed map; it provides the structure, insight, and direction to move forward purposefully.

Even fit individuals must find what works for their body. Professional bodybuilders and elite athletes don't all train the same, even with foundational moves like push-ups, pull-ups, squats, deadlifts, and bench presses. Trainers are hired not because athletes don't know how to train, but because the right trainer understands how to tailor programs to individual bodies, goals, and sports. Success depends on tweaking the details.

Michael Jordan's talent was immense; Tim Grover, in his book *Relentless*, unlocked his next level by customizing workouts to his physical and mental goals, evolving them over 15 years and six NBA championships. Greatness benefits from the right coach. It's about personalized guidance, learned through experience and observation—some lessons can only be taught in person, through movement, correction, and shared understanding.

Where Purpose Meets Precision

Fitness isn't a race against others—it's a return to self. It's the reclaiming of strength, control, and clarity through movement. While social media may celebrate extremes, true transformation is rooted in thoughtful action. Intelligent training is about discipline with direction—a measured pursuit that honors where you are while leading you to where you want to be.

Never Be Easy On Yourself

Consistency, The Cornerstone of Progress

Progress doesn't come from lifting the heaviest weights or chasing sweat-drenched exhaustion. It comes from showing up—again and again—with intention. Consistency, even in modified form, outpaces reckless intensity.

- **Modifications aren't signs of weakness.** They're adaptive tools, rooted in wisdom.

- Whether due to injury, age, or daily variability, adjusting your movement allows you to stay in the game and avoid unnecessary setbacks.

Consistency > Intensity.
Modifications ≠ Regression.
Effort is relative, not competitive.
Focus on your lane—your effort, your journey.

Training Adapted To You

Not Every Workout Plan Fits Every Body. A well-designed program must respect the individual—your history, your limitations, and your goals. Cookie-cutter plans overlook the nuances that matter: injury history, mobility, energy levels, recovery speed.

Your job is to find your **"Goldilocks Zone"**—that space where intensity meets safety, where the body is challenged but not punished. Sustainable training doesn't flirt with injury; it flirts with growth—patiently and persistently.

Modify With Intention

Adapt, Don't Abdicate

Modifications aren't about making exercises easier. They're about making them smarter and safer. You're not watering down your workout—you're reinforcing it.

When modifying:

- **Ask why.** Is it for safety, recovery, or better muscle engagement?

- **Keep the purpose.** The goal isn't comfort—it's control.

- **Build forward.** A good modification moves you closer to the full movement, if and when that's appropriate for your body. Know when to substitute. Always consult a seasoned professional.

Progress With Purpose

Not Every Day is Max Effort

There are days to push—and days to protect. Learn to read your body. Overtraining won't speed results; it only sets you back.

When recovery calls:
- You can try dropping the weight 20–30%
- Modify movement patterns
- Shift from volume to quality
- Emphasize activation and intention

This isn't slacking—it's strategy. Every choice you make in training is a vote for longevity or burnout.

Every Repetition is a Declaration

Move like it matters—because it does. Don't just go through the motions. Grip the weight. Breath with purpose. Contract the muscles. Control the descent.

- Full engagement over autopilot
- Precision over momentum
- Awareness over distraction

This is intelligent training:
Structured, yet adaptable.
Demanding, yet sustainable.
Simple—not easy.

You don't need to be the strongest or the fastest. You just need to show up—to dare, to try, to sweat, and to keep going. That's what matters. That's what changes lives. *As Theodore Roosevelt once said:*

As 2 Corinthians 10:5 says, "Bring every thought into captivity."

Fitness Became More Than a Routine, It Became Sacred

It touched every part of me—mental, emotional, spiritual. I started to see my body as a temple—worthy of nourishment, challenge, protection, and healing. The internal chaos began to settle. This wasn't just about survival. This was medicine. This was power.

I trained with all my heart because it mattered so much to me. Each healthy meal, early workout, and proud repetition felt like a small act of bravery, helping me face my fears. My muscles weren't just for show—they became a shield, protecting my mind from anxiety and doubt, and helping me feel stronger and more confident every day.

But the most profound change wasn't physical. It was a shift in my faith—believing I wasn't a mistake and that my past didn't define me. Perhaps that same unseen force, which once saved me from drowning years ago, still accompanied me—more strong than the bullies, louder than the fear, and deeper than the wounds.

> **Movement. Nourishment. Prayer. These weren't merely habits; they were vital lifelines—sacred, life-giving, and essential.**
>
> **Faith became my anchor. Discipline, my foundation. Fitness, my new language—a way of life.**

Over time, I realized that my trauma hadn't completely gone away—it had just shifted. The good news was, it no longer held power over me. That was my biggest breakthrough. With patience, discipline, and a sense of surrender, I managed to finally claim my mind. I began aligning my thoughts more closely with God's truth. Gradually, the old layers started to peel away, and a new, brighter version of myself began to come into view—more focused, stronger, and finally free.

I built up what I thought was beyond repair. The old story—the one that labeled me weak—I rewrote it. I rose from the ashes and took a deep, healing breath.

I spent years weighed down by my past—emotional pain, fears, doubts. I tried to heal with books, affirmations, and quick motivation. True healing happened when I finally let go—not as a sign of weakness, but as an act of trust. That was when I stopped trying to control everything and began leaning on something greater.

Transformation isn't just a one-time event. It's a decision you make over and over. And strength? It's not measured by how often you fall—it's measured by how often you get back up.

Everyone has flaws—shaped by pain and pride. But we're not meant to remain broken. True strength starts when we choose to change. Fear tried to shrink me, silence me, and make me disappear. Yet I learned: failure isn't the end. Regeneration was just one decision away.

And this transformation? It didn't just touch my body. It changed my spirit. I used to feel invisible—stuck in the shadows, misunderstood. But that story changed. I decided to shrink my circle and surround myself with people of purpose. People with depth, conviction, and integrity.

The boy who once hid in the background grew into a man who walked with quiet strength. Those years of loneliness weren't wasted; they were sacred and served as preparation.

"I am still as strong today as the day Moses sent me out; I'm just as vigorous to go out to battle now as I was then." — Joshua 14:11

"Praise the Lord, who is my rock. He trains my hands for war and gives my fingers skill for battle." — Psalm 144:1

Life Is Fleeting

My friend, I have made many mistakes, some of which weigh heavily on my heart, and some I wish I could undo. I've let down family, friends, and those who mattered most to me. **My journey through fitness was an awakening**, a lifeline that pulled me from the edge of destruction and reshaped me into a stronger, better version of myself. It healed so much—the social phobia, my insecurities, the deep wounds I carried, but even with that transformation, I still made mistakes in my marriage, family, and business.

Remember this: No matter how much you change or grow, you will always be human. You will still stumble and falter. Turning your life around—eating well, exercising, and striving to improve—does not make you immune to failure. Sometimes, those failures can be devastating. **That is why we must cherish every moment, every person, and** every fleeting second we are given, because in the end, it is not perfection that defines us, but the love we offer, the gratitude we show, and the way we honor those who walk this path with us.

> Be quick to forgive and express gratitude. Hold tightly to the people who support you and never take them for granted. The greatest regret lies not so much in our mistakes but in the love we fail to give when we still have the chance. The greatest gift you can give anyone, is the gift of your attention.

Time is a relentless thief, stealing moments we can never reclaim, it does not pause for regret, nor does it grant second chances; each fleeting opportunity, each unspoken word, drifts away like a pebble in the current, gone forever. I look back and feel their weight, not only as sorrow but also as lessons carved deep into my soul.

So, I urge you, do not chase hollow ambitions while the people who matter wait in the shadows of your neglect. Titles, possessions, fleeting success—none will love you back. They will not hold you in your weakest moments or remind you of your worth when the world feels unkind. Only the love we give, the bonds we nurture, will endure. Treasure them. Guard them fiercely because tomorrow is never promised.

No wealth is greater than the time spent with those who genuinely know and love you. No achievement replaces shared laughter, and no fortune equals the quiet comfort of an unspoken understanding. Yet we often fail to grasp their worth until they slip beyond reach. And by then, it is too late.

So, give your time freely. Love without hesitation. Offer kindness without expectation. These are the true legacies we leave behind—not wealth or status, but the moments we choose to be fully present.

The past cannot be rewritten, but it can teach us. It is not our prison—unless we make it so. What truly matters is now. This breath. This moment. The choices you make today will shape the story you leave behind. *Will you allow another day to slip away, lost to distractions that will never fulfill you? Or will you embrace today with open hands and an open heart, with the urgency of someone who understands just how fleeting it all is?* Let us not waste another second. Let us mend what is broken, reconnect with those we've neglected, and love without restraint.

> Because in the end, the greatest gift we can ever give is not riches, not words, but the undivided, irreplaceable gift of our attention.

Quotes That Carved My Path

Personal Growth & Mindset

To live strong with a good heart is to master the balance between resilience and compassion. It means being a warrior in life's battles—standing firm with unshakable strength while nurturing calm and kindness within; strength isn't found solely in the body, it lives in the discipline to persist, the courage to face what others cannot, and the perseverance to rise each time life knocks you down. But even deeper, real power resides in the heart—in the ability to uplift others, to show empathy in the midst of pain, and to extend grace even when the world offers none. This way of living shines brightest in adversity; it reveals that toughness doesn't require shutting down, and that gentleness is not weakness—it is wisdom. Through integrity, humility, and self-awareness, we don't merely endure; we evolve. We become warriors of peace, drawing our greatest strength not from how fiercely we fight, but from how deeply we care. A true warrior also shapes the mind into a tool for creativity, hope, and renewal—refusing to be defined by the weight of the past. They understand that thoughts shape habits, habits shape reality, and reality shapes life.

As Scripture teaches, **the renewing of the mind transforms destructive patterns into purposeful pathways filled with light.** A warrior's mindset rejects limitation and embraces possibility, seeing not narrow choices, but infinite horizons. **The warrior confronts fear, doubt, and anger—not by yielding, but by rising in faith, hope, and love.** Through that choice, life no longer appears as a wall of obstacles, but as a wide horizon of possibilities. By shaping the mind, the warrior shapes their reality—and in doing so, they become a living example of strength guided by compassion, and power led by purpose. What do you see when you look to the future? **The warrior envisions a world transformed by faith, hope, and love. Cultivate a warrior mindset.** – *The Author, Waldimir (Wally) B.*

- **Faith** anchors us to unseen futures, **hope** transforms every limitation into a doorway, **love** aligns us with a divine purpose; together, they expand the imagination, inspire perseverance, and enrich the soul's meaning. – Wally B.

- No weight of guilt can rewrite the past, nor can the grip of worry bend the future to your will. Yet, by surrendering to the present—with courage and purpose—you reclaim the only moment that truly belongs to you.

- Wherever you are, be there; don't be somewhere else. -Jim Rohn

- "Wisdom is applying knowledge. Without action, even a knowledgeable person is like an 'armchair philosopher.' Use your talents and be proactive." – Wally B.

- "Reaffirm your purpose daily to build discipline. If you falter, restart; this commitment can lead to meaningful changes in your life." – Wally B.

- When discipline becomes a habit, you may find yourself feeling more invigorated. Taking control of your decisions and dedicating yourself to your goals can weave discipline into the fabric of who you are. Embrace this journey to unlock your full potential." – Wally B.

- "To have what you want, you must first be who you truly are." – Wally B.

- "It's not just about overcoming problems, but what you become through them. Are you bitter or better?" – Wally B.

- "All the water in the ocean can't sink a ship unless it gets inside. Troubles can't sink you unless you let them in."

- "It's never too late to be who you might've been." -George Eliot

- "To waste time is to waste life; time is what life is made of." - Proverbial

- If you constantly feel busy, it's either a choice you made or one others made for you." – Wally B.

- "Yesterday is a voided check, tomorrow a promise of funds. Today is your only cash, so use it wisely." - Author Unknown

- "Some dream of a pool, while others barely use theirs. Some mourn lost loved ones, while others take theirs for granted. The hungry would give anything for a meal, while the full complain about the taste. The key? Gratitude. Someone, somewhere, would give everything for what you already have." - Hiroyuki Sanada, famed martial artist and actor

- "Take passionate action on your endeavor." -Wally B

- We are slowed more by the grain of sand in our shoe than the mountain we climb. – Muhammad Ali

- **The greatest gift you can give of yourself is "The gift of your attention."** -Wally B.

- Power of words: **"Your faith will never rise above the words of your mouth"**.

- A curve in the road is not the end of the road unless you fail to make the turn. -Helen Keller

- Embrace each new day, for it offers time—essential to life! Yesterday is an image, tomorrow a vision. Live your days well to turn yesterday into happiness and tomorrow into hope.

- What you become matters more than what you get. It's not, "What am I getting?" It should be, "What am I becoming?" This shapes you into the person you ultimately become. – Jim Rohn

- Your growth significantly impacts your accomplishments. -Wally B.

- If a picture paints a thousand words, then a few perfectly written words paint a thousand images/pictures. – Wally B.

- If I were everything I was called to be, how much better would the people around me be? -Wally B

- "And one last thing, friends: focus your thoughts on what's true, good, right, pure, beautiful, and worth respect. Think about what's excellent and worth praising." – Adapted from Phil. 4:8

- **The credit belongs to the one who is in the arena—who strives, who falls short, yet dares greatly—because even in failure, they stand apart from those who never risked at all.**
  — *Adapted from Theodore Roosevelt*

Overcoming Adversity

- "Everything is impossible until we actually do it. We all couldn't walk or do a push-up until we decided nothing will stop us." – Wally B.

- "Difficulties break some men but make others." – Nelson Mandela

- "We must all suffer one of two things: the pain of discipline or the pain of regret." – Jim Rohn

- "Whatever you don't hate, you will tolerate."

- "Determine that today you will overcome yourself of yesterday. Tomorrow, you will win over those of lesser skill, and later, over those of greater skill."

- "Truth is not what you want it to be. It is what it is, and you must bend to its power or live a lie." -Miyamoto Musashi

- "In fighting and in everyday life, you should be determined yet calm." --Miyamoto Musashi

- "You can't wait until life isn't hard anymore before you decide to be happy." - Nightbirde

Strength, Wisdom & Life Lessons

- "Caleb at 85: 'I'm as strong now as when Moses sent us on that journey, and I can still fight as well as I could then!" – Joshua 14:11

- 'Worrying is carrying tomorrow's load with today's strength—moving into tomorrow ahead of time. Worrying doesn't empty tomorrow of sorrow; it empties today of strength." – "Corrie Ten Boom

- "Make each day your masterpiece." – John Wooden

- You can get everything you want if you help enough people get what they want." – "Zig Ziglar

- 'Justice without power is empty; power without justice is violence." – "Musashi Miyamoto

- 'Ability is what you're capable of. Motivation determines what you do. Attitude determines how well you do it." – "Lou Holtz

- 'Youth is not a time of life; it is a state of mind. People grow old by deserting their ideals. You are as young as your faith, as old as your doubts; as young as your confidence, as old as your fears." – "Douglas MacArthur

- 'I'm as old as I've ever been, but I'm as young as I'll ever be." – "Robert O'Neal

Which map are you looking at? There is a paradigm of thinking that affects us all. You can look at a map of Illinois with all due diligence with five PhDs, but if you are trying to find Orlando, Florida, and all you have is an Illinois map, you will never find it because it is not there. You have the wrong map/ the wrong plan for your goal. So be sure that they are right when you seek your goals. – *A*dapted from Stephen R. Covey, The 7 Habits of Highly Effective People

One Day at A Time

There are two days each week in which we should not worry, nor let fear speak. Two days that must be kept free from despair, from doubt and burdens too heavy to bear.

One of these days is YESTERDAY. With its mistakes, its faults, its pain, its cares and blunders, its aches and sorrow, a past beyond our reach tomorrow. Yesterday has passed, forever beyond control, no wealth can change it, no power console, no act undone, no words erased, Yesterday's steps cannot be retraced.

The other day we should not fear, is TOMORROW with its burdens near, its promises large, its failures unknown, future beyond what today has shown. Tomorrow's sun will rise once more, in golden light or clouds that pour. But rise it will, beyond our sway, for tomorrow is not ours today.

This leaves but one day; TODAY! Any person can fight the battle of just one day, it is only when you have the burdens of those two other entities yesterday and tomorrow that we breakdown. It's not the experiences of today that drive us mad, it's remorse and bitterness for something which happened yesterday and the dread of what tomorrow may bring. Let us therefore live one day at a time. - *Dr. Robert Burdette*

No "Buts" About It

"But" is a frightening word. It signals an excuse. This three-letter word can kill a thought that starts with "do it." To get what we want, we first have to know what we want.

Then, we must figure out what to do to achieve it. Finally, we have to make the time to do it. In other words, we need the means and the opportunity. When all is in place, we say "But," stopping ourselves. Instead of gaining experience and achieving goals, we accept excuses. This word halts progress, making us reason why we can't try. It's astounding how a three-letter word holds us back.

"But" represents fear—fear that we'll look foolish, fear of rejection, fear that we won't succeed, fear that we *can't* do it, or just general fear of the unknown. Whatever the fear, it can be devastating, stopping us from reaching our goals. We often use "but" to delay action. We should act now, but we convince ourselves tomorrow we'll feel better. Good intentions are easily postponed, and "but" provides a rationalization for our excuses.

We justify inaction with patience, claiming good things take time and waiting will be better. We delay decision-making, but as we dwell on excuses, time slips away—time we can never regain.

Life is either used for *living* or for *excuses*. *"But"* starts the excuses. *"Do it"* starts the living.

Next time you hear the word *"but,"* be on guard. Say to yourself, *"No buts for me,"* and do what you were about to do.

Remember, Henry Ford said, *"I'm going to build an automobile."* And George Flamish said, *"But."* We all know who Henry Ford is. Nobody knows George Flamish.

Get the point? No *"buts"* about it. **After all is said and done, more is said than done.** — Adapted from Aaron R. Fodiman

Discipline & Motivation

- "Daily actions matter. Like consistently chopping a mighty oak, small efforts lead to progress. Time and persistence are essential for achieving goals."

- "Use today wisely for growth and meaningful experiences. Strive for success and avoid regrets. Failure only occurs if you stop trying."

- "Don't dwell on past regrets: use mistakes as learning experiences."

- "Practice until you can't get it wrong."

- "It's okay to be sure of yourself—you have no choice; nobody else will."

- "It is not what you do that makes you who you are. It is who you are that makes you do what you do." – unknown

- "Discipline is the bridge between goals and accomplishments." -Jim Rohn

- "Motivation gets you started, but purpose keeps you going."

- "Don't let fatigue make a coward of you." – Wally B.

- "You are not defeated when you lose; you are defeated when you quit."

- Fortify your mind to empower an unstoppable body.

- "Life is a grindstone. Whether it grinds you down or polishes you up depends on what you are made of. A stone without density falls apart and turns to powder, while a gemstone becomes more valuable when it is ground. What are you made of? Be assured—you are a gem, a diamond in the making!" — Jacob M. Braude

- Please don't wait for that proverbial ship to come because it probably won't. You build the ship and sail it to where YOU want to go!

- **Just one second:** Quitting takes just a second—just one moment to say, "I'm done." Yet that exact moment can lead to your breakthrough. Whenever you consider giving up on your workout, goal, or dream, take a pause. That split-second decision influences everything. Choose to push forward. Reject the urge to back down. A single second is all it requires to transform your life—and that choice is always yours. – Wally B.

- **A question to one's commitment when put to a vital test:** "Will you now stop at only words when you are needed most? Is that the sort of person you are? "I ask only that you act upon the beliefs of which you have so strongly spoken and in which you so strongly believe". – Wally B.

Chapter 3
FITNESS GUIDELINES

Resistance Training

Resistance training isn't just about gaining size—it's about developing **muscle *density***, improving strength, and **boosting your metabolis**m. Whether you're using machines, free weights, or your own body weight, resistance training is essential, even push-ups count as resistance training, because you're pushing your own body weight (roughly 65%).

The right approach depends on your background, goals, and physical condition. These ***general* rep ranges** can provide helpful guidance:

- 8 to 12 reps: strength and hypertrophy

- 12 to 15+ reps targets muscular endurance, and yes, you can still build size in this range. There are many solid, proven training methods; some debated, others widely accepted.

- As I've said before, we're all different. The most important thing is to find what works best for you.

- Aim for at least 3 sets of each exercise, performed several days a week. Be sure to adjust your training volume and frequency based on your recovery, experience level, and overall training history.

- A personalized approach always delivers the best results.

Experiment and Document Your Progress:
Each training session is a chance to learn what works best for your body. Keep a dedicated notebook or digital log and record **every detail**: the type of exercise, whether you're using machines or free weights, the exact weight used, reps, sets, and how you felt during the workout. This habit builds awareness, tracks progress, and helps you make smart adjustments. **Include your weight, measurements, diet, vitamins, how you're sleeping, etc.**

> Over time, patterns will emerge—**what challenges you, what leads to plateaus, and what drives results**. Use this information to tweak your routine. Don't be afraid to experiment with different equipment, tempos, or rest periods. Modify exercises as needed, but always track what you change and why. This isn't just about lifting—it's about building a personalized, evolving blueprint for your success.

Circuit Training and HIIT: Efficient & Effective

For overall fitness and fat loss, **circuit training** is one of the most effective methods. It involves cycling through different exercises—like machines, dumbbells, push-ups, and pull-ups—with little rest in between.

HIIT (High-Intensity Interval Training) is another excellent approach. It combines short bursts of effort with brief rest periods and often includes:

- Bodyweight exercises like air squats, push-ups, and pull-ups
- Dumbbells, kettlebells, or machine-based resistance movements

Workouts typically last 30 to 45 minutes. If your fitness level allows it keep intensity around Level 2 on standard exertion charts (easily found online) for the best results.

Weightlifting & Cardio: Best Sequence for Fat Burn

"If your routine focuses on weight training—lat pulldowns, rows, bench presses, deadlifts, squats, or dumbbell work—you're in the traditional resistance training zone."

For optimal fat burning, it's most effective to perform cardio *after* your strength workout. At that point, your body has likely used much of its glycogen (carbohydrate) stores, making it more likely to tap into fat as a fuel source during a 20-minute cardio session.

However, if you're doing **HIIT (High-Intensity Interval Training)**, there's no need to add extra cardio afterward. HIIT combines both resistance and cardiovascular elements, providing a comprehensive fat-burning workout on its own.

Foundational Movements That Deliver Results: Throughout this book, I've emphasized the importance of effective foundational movements. Exercises like **push-ups**, **squats**, and **pull-ups**—even with assistance from bands or machines—are consistently excellent choices.

When performing squats, placing the bar across your **upper back and traps** is one of the most powerful techniques. This approach is typically best for those who are already well-conditioned. However, it's important to be mindful of **spinal compression**. That's why I often recommend **leg press machines**—though not all are created equal. Some designs may place stress on the lower back, so be sure the **ergonomics** are correct.

Hack squat machines are another great option. The seated (compact) versions with long back pads provide support and reduce spinal loading. Even standing hack machines that rest on your shoulders are usually safer than placing a heavy bar directly across your neck.

"In military boot camp, recruits arrive in all shapes—some overweight, some underweight. After 8–10 weeks, most are lean and fit. Why? Because training emphasizes full-body exercise and endurance. Build your base with legs, back, and chest strength. Once the foundation is solid, refine smaller muscles like biceps, triceps, and shoulders. That's the shift from getting in shape to sculpting the body you want."

Exercises for Runners

1. Consider Your Starting Point

General Fitness: These tips are suitable for individuals in good shape without significant injuries or chronic issues. If you have concerns, like bad knees or joint problems, consult a qualified trainer or healthcare professional to tailor your training accordingly.

Age and Ability: While younger runners may recover more quickly, adults in their 40s, 50s, and older can also benefit from these techniques *when adapted to your needs*.

2. Understand Your Training Goals

Are you training for a flat race, hilly terrain, or trail running? The type of terrain determines the focus of your workouts. For example, trail runners require agility and coordination, while road runners prioritize speed and endurance.

3. Incorporate Plyometric Training

What Are Plyometrics? Plyometric exercises (to increase measure) focus on explosive movements that boost power and agility. These include box jumps, long jumps, and lateral hops. Plyometrics enhance reactive strength and improve runners' agility, which is crucial.

How to Do It Safely:

- Start with low box heights (6–12 inches or whatever you know you're comfortable with).

- Progress gradually as you build strength and confidence.

- Work with a knowledgeable trainer to ensure proper form and prevent injury; many are attempting 36 to 42+ inch box jumps, most aren't athletes—they're everyday gym-goers, in my opinion, that's often uncalled for.

- Box jumps can be effective, but only **when used correctly**. Without proper conditioning and gradual progression, it can lead to serious shin and knee injuries, unless you're training for a sport like **basketball or volleyball, where vertical jump matters**, there's *rarely* a need to jump much higher than 24 inches.

- **Every exercise should have a purpose.** Doing something just because everyone else is doing it isn't reason enough. **Train smart, not flashy.**

- Keep this in mind during jumps: **Land softly.** I refer to it as "soft knees." Imagine you're landing on rice paper—you want to make very little noise when you touch down. This technique reduces stress on your knees and helps you become lighter on your feet, which is crucial and often overlooked by many. Plyometrics can help reduce the risk of injury when navigating obstacles like curbs, roots, or uneven terrain by making you more agile.

4. Upgrade Your Body's Engine – Hot Rod Blower: A blower is a type of supercharger that forces more air into the engine's intake, allowing more fuel to burn. This boosts horsepower by increasing the air-fuel mixture the engine can use, resulting in more powerful combustion.

- **Focus on Aerobic Capacity (VO_2 Max):** VO_2 max is your body's ability to use oxygen efficiently during exercise. It reflects how well your heart, lungs, and muscles work together to sustain activity. The higher your VO_2 max, the better your endurance and overall performance.

- **Why It Matters:** VO_2 (volume of oxygen) measures how many liters of oxygen your body uses per minute. It's a key indicator of aerobic fitness and cardiovascular efficiency—showing how much oxygen your body can take in, transport, and use during exertion.

5. Include Sprint Training

Sprint intervals improve your speed, endurance, and running economy. Schedule 1–2 sprints weekly, emphasizing short bursts (20–60 seconds) with recovery in between. **Try this if you're fit enough:**

> Mark Spitz, the legendary swimmer who won seven gold medals at the 1972 Munich Olympics, trained under Coach Doc Counsilman, who believed in the power of **overtraining** *[of a different sort]*. Doc had Spitz consistently swim longer distances in practice than he would in competition, building endurance, confidence, and mental grit. So if you're gearing up for a race—say a 5K—consider stretching your training runs to 7k or even 10K. ***Pushing just past your goal distance in training might be the edge you need on race day.***

6. Stretching and Recovery

- Before running, perform a brief *dynamic* warm-up and stretch to activate your muscles and improve mobility.

- After Running: *Static* stretch thoroughly to prevent tightness and reduce cramping. Target key muscle groups like hamstrings, calves, quads, and hip flexors.

7. Long-Term Considerations
- Consistency Over Time: Avoid falling for short-term trends or one-size-fits-all advice. Your training plan should evolve based on your goals, fitness level, and experience.
- Balance: Mix your running routine with cross-training (e.g., strength training or cycling) to reduce the risk of overuse injuries and enhance overall performance.

8. Effort Is Key

No magic pill or perfect plan can replace effort, discipline, and consistency. Whether you're running for fun or training for a marathon, success comes from your commitment to put in the work.

Running is more than just putting one foot in front of the other—it's a balance of training, discipline, and self-care. Your body is your most valuable asset, so take care of it with proper training, nutrition, and recovery.

My Fitness Principles

- Never drink water in the middle of a set; wait till the end of the circuit, set, or round.

- During a HIIT or Circuit routine, between exercises, rest just enough to "Catch your breath" - then a 90-120 sec. recovery (if in good physical condition, that *may* be enough).

- Do not converse while you're in the midst of an exercise.

- The gym can be friendly, but it exists for training, not overly socializing.

- **You shall always firmly engage/contract your abdominal muscles during most exercises, when practical.**

- Do not train when under-fueled or overly full.

- **Always control your breathing.**

- **Focused muscle contraction maximizes results.**

- Consistency, intensity, proper form, and diet are major keys to fitness success.

- "If you let life get in the way of your fitness, then your health will get in the way of your life."

- **"NEVER enter a gym without a planned routine. Success = Planning!"**

- **When you give your full, honest effort in a workout and leave feeling accomplished, that's success.**

- "If exercise is uncomfortable, how uncomfortable is carrying extra weight and its issues (back pain, diabetes, etc.)?

- Abdominal strength is built through training; visibility depends largely on nutrition and body composition.

- "It is exercise alone that supports the spirit and keeps the mind in vigor." – "Marcus Tullius Cicero

- "Lack of activity destroys the good condition of every human, while movement & physical exercise save it and preserve it." – Plato

- "Our health always seems much more valuable after we lose it."

- **"It is not the exercise that works you; it's YOU that must work the exercise."**

- **Visualize the muscle group before a set. Proper form begins in the mind.**

- **Sacrifice bad habits to become your best.**

- The best training partner a person can have, in my opinion, is the clock.

- "You don't have to love the workouts, but you can crave the results."

- Overeating is when your tongue writes checks that your body cannot cash.

- "It's not necessarily what you eat that leads to an early grave—it's what eats at you."

- Everyone enjoys the experience of driving in a newer vehicle. Just as people feel more confident in nice clothes, why not treat yourself to a fresh new "skin"?

- A few simple disciplines repeated every day.

- **Perform each repetition with intent and control.**

By meal planning/prepping, you rely on willpower once a week. In contrast, you face 21 potentially poor food choices each week without it.

Mistakes Made at the Gym

1. Not Focusing on the Basics

One of the biggest mistakes people make at the gym is overcomplicating their workouts with fancy techniques or trends. While many modern workout methods and equipment are available, it is essential to often stick to the basics. Effective workouts come down to **proper form and consistency, not flashy moves.** Focus on simple, **foundational exercises that effectively target your muscles.**

2. Too Much Talking

Talking too much while working out is a common mistake at the gym. Conversation can interrupt your workout flow and diminish the intensity of your training. You're not maximizing your performance if you're talking excessively rather than concentrating on your workouts. **Use the clock as your training partner to help you stay on track and manage your rest periods.**

Keep track of your rest times, whether 45 seconds or 3 minutes, and use them efficiently. During your rest time, concentrate on what you just accomplished and focus on your next exercise, visualizing the movement in your mind so you have a better mind-muscle connection.

3. Lack of Focus on Form and Technique: Proper form is essential for every exercise. The technique should always come before the number of reps, whether you're doing squats, presses, or any other movement. **Reaching A Specific Rep Count May Feel Satisfying, But Poor Form Can Lead To Injury And Reduce Workout Effectiveness. Always Prioritize Activating The Correct Muscles, Maintaining Proper Posture, And Engaging Your Core With Every Movement.** Remember, *perfect practice makes perfect*, not just doing the reps to hit a number.

4. Setting Unrealistic Expectations for Reps and Progress. Many people become fixated on achieving specific repetitions, such as aiming for 12, even when difficult. The focus should be on challenging yourself with **the correct form rather than just reaching a target number**. If you're having trouble completing the recommended number of reps with proper form, it may be time to reevaluate your weight or the rep count. Striving for proper technique and muscle engagement is far more valuable than rushing to complete a set. Always prioritize quality over quantity.

5. Not Engaging the Right Muscles

When exercising, it's crucial to ensure you're engaging the correct muscle groups. Mind-muscle connection is key to building strength and muscle tone. Whether it's a squat, deadlift, or bench press, focus on making each movement count. If your movements aren't engaging the right muscles, you're not maximizing the benefit of the exercise. Stay mindful of your body's alignment and actively engage your core, glutes, or other key muscle groups during these movement.

6. Too Much Running Around and Phone Usage. Spending excessive time on your phone or switching between different machines *unnecessarily* results in a disorganized workout. Stay committed to your plan. If you regularly pause to check your phone or engage in conversations, you're not training with sufficient intensity. Maintain efficient rest periods and concentrate on the task at hand to optimize your workout results.

The Importance of Consistency and Focus – the key to seeing real progress: Work hard and follow the plan you've set for yourself. Concentrate on your exercises and ensure you're giving your best effort safely and effectively. Remember, it's not about random workouts or distractions; it's about working with purpose, engaging muscles properly, and pushing yourself—*safely*.

Goal Met, Now What?

1. You Don't Have to Push Beyond Your Goals

Once you reach your fitness goals, focusing on maintaining your progress is perfectly fine. Many people must keep pushing harder, but this isn't necessary unless your goals evolve. Maintenance is about consistency, not intensity.

Key points:

- You don't need to train like an Olympic athlete.

- Pushing yourself to exhaustion or vomiting after workouts is not healthy or productive.

- Overtraining can lead to unnecessary strain and injury.

2. Training Intensity: What's Right for You?

> Exercising doesn't need to leave you exhausted or crawling out of the gym. The key is moderation and purpose. Professional athletes may train for many hours a day, but what's often overlooked is how they manage intensity. They work within their lactate threshold—stopping before significant lactic acid buildup. They also rotate training types, focusing at different times on power, agility, speed, plyometrics, or technique. By varying focus and allowing recovery between muscle groups or energy systems, they can sustain long training sessions without breaking down.

Lactate Threshold: Training within your limits helps prevent muscle fatigue and burnout. Athletes may push these boundaries strategically, but moderate efforts are effective for most people.

Avoid high-risk movements like advanced Olympic lifts (clean and jerk, snatches) **unless you are specifically trained in them**. They are unnecessary and unsafe for the *average* person.

3. Maintenance Training for Longevity

If you've reached your goals, here's one good way to maintain your fitness:

- Frequency: 2–3 sessions per week are sufficient.

- Duration: 30–60 minutes per session.

- Intensity: Moderate. Avoid training to failure unless you have a specific reason, like preparing for a sport.

- Rest Between Sets: 1–3 minutes, depending on the exercise, weight, and intensity.

Tips:
- Stick to the proper weight or resistance levels until you feel ready to adjust.

- Change reps or sets occasionally to keep things engaging.

Focus on movements that support *functional* fitness, especially as you age.

4. Reps and Sets: General Guidelines
To Maintain Strength and Health

Reps: 8–15 per set, adjusted to your fitness level and goals

Sets per Session: 3–5 per body part

Weekly Volume: 10–20 total sets per body part, which is sufficient for most people.

5. Specific Exercises to Maintain Fitness
Weight Training: Machines, dumbbells, resistance bands, or bodyweight exercises. Machines with *adjustable angles* are ideal for joint health.

- Aerobics: Moderate-intensity cardio helps maintain cardiovascular health.

- Functional Movements: Exercises that mimic real-life activities, like bodyweight squats or light kettlebell deadlifts, help improve mobility and strength.

6. Safety and Adaptability
- Avoid extreme weights or risky movements as you age.

- Support your form with machines or props when needed.

- If you like box jumps, modify the height to lessen joint strain and focus on landing softly—think soft knees, as if landing on rice paper.

7. Nutrition for Maintenance – See Nutrition Section
Fitness is only one part of the equation; nutrition is vital to maintaining progress. **80% of weight loss is nutrition.**

- Protein: Maintain adequate intake to support muscle recovery.

- Carbohydrates: Focus on complex carbs for energy.

- Fats: Choose healthy fats while minimizing trans and saturated fats.

- Sodium: Keep your intake in check, especially if you have high blood pressure.

Maintenance is about consistently performing your activities over time. You don't need to increase intensity or volume continually. Instead, prioritize injury prevention and overall well-being.

> **Summary:** After reaching fitness goals, avoid constant overexertion. Maintenance involves balancing health and lifestyle without overtraining. Follow a structured plan, listen to your body, **rest as needed**, and manage nutrition. Consistency helps you enjoy fitness benefits long term.

Chapter 4
EFFECTIVE WORKOUT PLANS

Choose Your Approach

This book is designed as a practical starting point for the average person seeking better health and fitness. With countless exercise variations and training philosophies available, it's important to understand that fitness is highly personal. What works well for one individual may not work for another. Factors such as age, ability, and personal goals all matter.

Because of this, no single program fits everyone. Trying to cover every possible training method in one book would require multiple volumes—and even then, it would fall short, as both the science and practical application of fitness continue to evolve.

My hope is that this book provides a solid foundation—drawn from decades of hands-on experience—to help you move forward with clarity, purpose, and confidence.

With over five decades in the fitness world, I don't claim to know everything. I have, however, been fortunate to gain a deep well of experience that allows me to guide and support others on their path. This book is not intended to serve as a complete training manual. Instead, it offers a thoughtful framework—principles and sample structures you can build upon with intention and clarity.

I've kept things basic here for good reason. Personalized fitness is best achieved through hands-on coaching. If you choose to research on your own, make sure your information comes from reputable, science-based sources—not trends or social media influencers.

Use this section as a compass, not a map. It won't give you every workout or variation, but it will give you a foundation. The goal is not to hand you a complete training system, but to show how fitness changed and saved my life—and to guide you with principles you can build on with confidence, whether at home or in the gym.

Finding What Works for You

There are many effective training methods—but success depends on choosing the one that aligns with your needs and applying it consistently.

Your selection should be based on:

- **Your current fitness level** (beginner, intermediate, or advanced)

- **Your primary objective** (strength, endurance, hypertrophy, fat loss, etc.)

- **Your recovery capacity** (some people thrive with higher volume, while others need more rest and lower frequency)

The right method is the one that challenges you appropriately, supports your goals, and respects your body's ability to adapt and recover.

Do What You Enjoy—But Make Sure It's Effective!

The key to long-term fitness is consistency, and consistency comes from enjoyment. You need a training style you actually look forward to—but it must also deliver results. The best path is one that's both enjoyable and effective, reshaping your body, strengthening your health, and building lasting strength.

Let's be clear: if your preferred activity is aerobic classes like Zumba or dance cardio, that's a positive starting point. These activities support heart health, coordination, movement, and energy. However, aerobic training alone is not enough to produce meaningful improvements in strength, posture, bone health, or overall body structure.

To truly change your body—by building lean muscle, supporting metabolism, and improving posture and structural strength—you need resistance training. That doesn't mean lifting recklessly or chasing exhaustion. It means using resistance that meaningfully challenges you within an appropriate repetition range—often somewhere between **8 and**

20 controlled repetitions, depending on the individual—while maintaining proper form. That range represents a common and effective foundation for strength training.

Muscle Density, Not Bulk

Strength training is often misunderstood. The goal is not bulk; it is density. Lean, strong muscle tissue improves how efficiently your body functions and uses energy, including at rest. Over time, this leads to a stronger, more resilient body and better long-term metabolic health.

The Ideal Formula? A Hybrid Approach

You don't have to choose one thing forever. Combine what you *love* with what your body needs:

- Love tennis? Great—add two functional resistance training sessions a week.
- Enjoy Zumba? Perfect—supplement it with a short but intense strength circuit.
- Like walking or jogging? Pair it with weighted movements or bodyweight training.

*This is how you build a sustainable, enjoyable, and **effective** routine.*

Bottom Line:

- Do what you enjoy—but make sure it supports your goals.
- Incorporate strength training—for structure, metabolism, and results.
- Challenge your muscles—don't just move; engage and strengthen.
- Your body needs resistance to change. Find your balance—but don't skip the strength.

Workout Styles to Explore

Mind-Body & Control-Based

- Yoga – Flexibility, breath, and mind-body connection
- Pilates – Core strength, posture, and control
- Tai Chi – Gentle movement, balance, and mental clarity

Strength & Conditioning
- Calisthenics – Bodyweight-based strength and mobility
- Resistance Training – Using bands or weights to build muscle
- Weight Training – Beginner, Intermediate, Advanced routines
- Bodybuilding – Muscle hypertrophy through structured programs

High Intensity & Functional
- HIIT (High-Intensity Interval Training) – Short bursts, high effort
- MIT (Moderate Intensity Training) – Sustained, manageable effort
- Circuit Training – Rotating exercises for full-body activation
- Boot Camp Classes – Group-based, high-intensity circuit training

Cardio & Endurance
- Swimming – Low-impact, full-body cardio and endurance
- Running/Jogging – Accessible cardiovascular training
- Cycling/Spin – Endurance and lower-body power
- Dance Fitness – Rhythmic cardio (e.g., Zumba, hip-hop)

Skill-Based & Athletic
- Martial Arts – Discipline, agility, and coordination

- Parkour – Urban agility, strength, and mobility

- Tennis/Pickleball – Sport-based cardio and quick reflexes

> **No Weight Should Feel Light, and No Move Should Feel Easy**

A Basic Well-Rounded Weekly Weightlifting Guide

- 2–4 days of resistance training: using dumbbells, bands, machines, or bodyweight.

- 1–2 days of mobility and core work: focusing on flexibility, stability, and posture.

- Optional cardio: walking, cycling, or circuits, added based on your goals.

Prioritize Progressive Overload—Safely:

Gradually increasing resistance is essential for improving strength, endurance, and overall fitness. This principle, known as progressive overload, allows the body to adapt and grow stronger over time—but it must be applied with intention and care.

There are countless variations of resistance training, and not every exercise is appropriate for every individual. The guidelines presented here are designed for those newer to structured training. When performed correctly and safely, these exercises serve as effective building blocks for long-term progress.

I strongly encourage you to continue learning—read, research, observe, and ask questions. Most importantly, seek guidance from experienced, knowledgeable trainers. There is no substitute for one-on-one instruction, especially when it comes to proper form, progression, and injury prevention.

> **While this book provides a solid foundation, it's impossible to cover every detail of every movement. Let this be your starting point, and let curiosity, consistency, good coaching and safety guide the rest.**

- Stick to the basics and avoid overcomplicating your routine.

- Avoid excessive talking and distractions; use the clock to manage rest periods.

- Prioritize proper form over hitting arbitrary rep numbers.

- **Engage the correct muscles in every exercise and focus on maintaining proper body alignment.**

- Be consistent, focused, and intentional with your workouts.

You don't need a complicated routine to get in shape.

A few well-chosen tools—a rower, a pull-up bar (using loop bands for assistance when needed), and push-ups—can cover most of what the body requires. If a pull-up bar isn't an option, resistance bands can be used effectively for back rows at low, mid, and high anchor points.

These types of exercises can train **70–80% of the body** by targeting major muscle groups that naturally involve the arms. For most people, there is no need to isolate biceps and triceps early on. When you train the back, you train the biceps. When you train the chest, you train the triceps—and the shoulders are involved in both. Once a person reaches a higher level of conditioning and functional fitness, focused arm work can be added if desired.

Relying heavily on isolated arm exercises too early—common in some group-class formats—burns relatively few calories and limits overall strength development, particularly through the core. While isolation has a place, it should not replace foundational movement patterns.

> **Compound Movements**
> Compound exercises are fundamental for improving strength, increasing muscle density, and enhancing metabolic efficiency. These movements involve multiple joints and muscle groups working together—such as squats, deadlifts, bench presses, rows, and pull-ups. This creates greater neuromuscular demand and a stronger systemic training effect than isolated exercises.

> Over time, compound training improves coordination, increases overall energy expenditure, and stimulates lean muscle development. The result is a stronger, more efficient body with a higher resting metabolic rate and better long-term fitness outcomes.

Rate of Perceived Exertion in Resistance Training

This particular format starts at five:

5: Fairly easy, like a warm-up weight.

6: You can perform 4-5 more repetitions.

7: You can manage 2-3 more reps.

8: You have 2 more left in the tank, and no more!

9: You have 1 more left in the tank, and no more!

10: Reach total muscle failure with perfect form.

11: Reach total muscle failure with loose form after completing perfect reps.

12: Use dynamic technique (some momentum) to push beyond failure; after 2-3 tries, you cannot move the weight.

My Take on Planks

Are Planks Good for Core Development?

Planks can be a **very effective starting exercise** for people who are beginning to get in shape. They teach basic core bracing, body awareness, and stability with minimal complexity. For individuals who are deconditioned or new to structured training, planks serve an important early role.

The limitation is that planks are a **static exercise**. While they help establish initial stability, most people perform them at relatively low intensity, which limits long-term core development. Sustaining meaningful, high-effort muscle engagement for extended periods is difficult unless the contraction is intentionally maximized. True high-effort isometric contractions typically fatigue within **10–30 seconds**, depending on the individual and the level of tension applied.

Because of this, planks should be viewed as a **stepping stone, not an endpoint**. When performed with high tension, isometric exercises fatigue quickly and often produce visible signs such as shaking, which reflects increased motor-unit recruitment. **This type of short-duration, high-tension isometric work has long been used in athletic and martial training systems.**

Progression Rule

When you can maintain a strong plank with full-body tension for **20–30 seconds**, it's time to progress to more dynamic core work.

Conclusion

Planks are valuable for building early core stability and awareness. As strength and control improve, however, greater benefits come from dynamic exercises that require the core to stabilize and transfer force through movement—such as push-ups, carries, and compound lifts. Training the core as part of integrated movement leads to better strength, coordination, and long-term functional progress than static holds alone.

Descending Ladders -A great challenge

If you are **more highly fit or working toward peak conditioning**, descending ladder and pyramid exercises can effectively challenge your muscular endurance, strength, and cardiovascular capacity. These training methods leverage progressive overload, metabolic stress, and neuromuscular adaptation, all contributing to improved fitness.

Descending ladder workouts involve starting with a high number of repetitions and decreasing with each subsequent set. For example, **start with 10, 12, or 15 reps for each, then decrease to 5 reps, completing just one round. 15 down to 5 = 110 reps for ea. one, X4 exercises = 440 total reps.** *modify by:* **12>5, or 10>5.**

Samples: You can pick and choose, switch these around, or come up with your own. Pick four exercises that you love. They're going to work your body. Especially on vacation when you have a short time, and it's fun; *(if you want to swap in a cardio move like jumping jacks or mountain climbers, just do the count or time. For jumping jacks, do 30–50 reps; for mountain climbers, go 30–60 seconds per round).*

- Push-ups

- Inverted Back Row

- Box jumps

or,

- TRX Squat & Row
- Weighted Walking Lunges [reps are each leg]
- Dumbell Curl, Squat with Overhead Press

Pyramid Pushups-Fun, but tough
- Progressive Fatigue Adaptation
- Time-Efficient: Maximizes muscle engagement in a short period.
- High Volume with Less Burnout: Allows for sustained intensity while managing muscle fatigue.

Pyramid workouts can be ascending, descending, or both (full). You can increase reps before reducing them, or increase resistance while lowering reps (or vice versa).

Example:
We often start at **30**, **40**, or even **50**, depending on fitness level.
30's: 30,20,10 / 20,30,10 =**120**

Physiological Benefits:
- Motor Unit Recruitment: Increasing resistance over time activates additional muscle fibers, enhancing strength.
- Metabolic Conditioning: Aids in fat burning and builds muscular endurance during longer exercise sessions.
- Enhanced Strength-Endurance Ratio: Develops both slow-twitch and fast-twitch muscle fibers.

Finding What Works for You
There are numerous training methods, all of which can be effective when used correctly. Your selection should be based on:
- Your current fitness level (beginner, intermediate, advanced)

- Your objective (strength, endurance, hypertrophy, fat loss, etc.)

- Your recovery capacity (some individuals may benefit from higher volume, while others may need less).

Athletes and Bodybuilders Have Different Training Approaches

- Some choose high volume (multiple sets, moderate weight) to achieve hypertrophy.

- Others concentrate on low volume with high-intensity strength training.

- Some prioritize negative (eccentric) training, which involves slowly lowering the weight to maximize muscle damage and promote growth.

Final Thought: Success Comes from Your Efforts.

> **Success isn't determined by the exercise itself, but by how you consistently and progressively implement it. There isn't one "best" method; the crucial factors are proper execution, intensity, and recovery.**

Action Steps:
- Begin at an appropriate intensity for your fitness level.

- Always perform a warm-up to prepare your muscles and joints.

- Experiment with different training styles to find what keeps you motivated and improving.

- Train with intention. Progress with consistency. Adapt as needed.

Chapter 5
IMPORTANCE OF RESISTANCE TRAINING

Proper Muscle Contraction – Key to Results

When it comes to working out, one critical element is often overlooked: **muscle contraction**. Many people fail to properly contract the muscles they're targeting, which minimizes the effectiveness of their training. Here's how to get it right.

Take the lat pulldown or most back row techniques. A common mistake is focusing on pulling the bar with your arms—driving the elbows as the first move—rather than **initiating the movement with your back muscles**. The latissimus dorsi is the primary muscle here. Whether you're doing a dumbbell back row, T-bar row, barbell row, or cable row, start by engaging the muscles around your shoulder blades; then drive the arms backfocusing on "crushing a walnut" between your shoulder blades. **Your arms should be like hooks to connect to whatever apparatus you're using, don't overwork them; let your back do the work - you'll feel the difference immediately when the focus is correct.**

Bicep Curls: Don't just lift and lower the weight—connect mentally with your biceps.

- Start by contracting the biceps, not swinging your arms.

- Squeeze hard at the top of each rep.

- Slowly lower the weight, maintaining control and tension.

Where This Applies: Use this mind-muscle connection approach in other exercises too—like dumbbell flies, back rows, leg extensions, and more. The more intentional your movement, the better your results.

Some Exceptions: Certain compound movements, like the flat barbell bench press, don't allow for full isolated contraction. That's okay. In those cases, just focus on good form, steady tempo, and a full range of motion.

Avoid Overtraining: Pushing your body too hard without adequate rest can lead to serious consequences. One rare but dangerous condition is **rhabdomyolysis**, where muscle tissue breaks down so severely it leaks into the bloodstream and can damage your kidneys. It's preventable—so respect recovery.

Train Smart: Learn proper technique. Rest enough. Stick with trusted sources for information. Avoid random fitness advice from people who lack the experience or credentials to back it up.

Training Principles To Live By

- Every Rep Counts: Be fully present in every rep. Focus on the muscles you're working on and give it your full attention. Mind your form and concentrate on the contraction for maximum results.

- Train Wisely, Not Recklessly: Push yourself, but don't risk injury. Use the intelligence and intuition you've been given.

- Balance and Recovery: Rest and recovery are just as important as the work you put in. Listen to your body and adjust as needed.

- "Rest As Much as You Have To But As Little as You Need To."

Muscle Memory

Muscle memory is a legitimate, science-backed process. It refers to the brain and body's ability to quickly regain physical skills and strength after a break in training. Whether you're a weightlifter returning post-injury or a stroke survivor retraining movement, muscle memory is a valuable ally.

What Is Muscle Memory? When we repeat a movement over time, such as lifting weights, typing, or walking, our brain develops neural pathways that make the movement more automatic. This process entails both the central nervous system and tangible changes in muscle cells.

Research indicates that muscles add nuclei (called myonuclear) to muscle fibers when they grow. These nuclei remain even after muscles shrink due to inactivity. When training resumes, these retained nuclei facilitate faster muscle regrowth—this is the biological basis of muscle memory.

How Long Does It Last? Muscle memory can last for months or even years. Studies have shown that individuals who trained for an extended period and then took months or years off regained muscle mass and strength much faster than first-time lifters.

- Short breaks (up to 3 months): Strength and skill return within a few weeks.

- Long breaks (years): Myonuclear remain embedded in the muscle fibers, facilitating quicker retraining, particularly if the person has trained consistently in the past.

"A study found that consistent, long-term lifters—serious trainees rather than occasional participants—who had detrained for ~15 years regained muscle substantially faster than individuals with very little training history." (Bruusgaard & Gundersen, *PNAS*, 2008)."

Why It Matters in Rehabilitation: Muscle memory serves as a lifeline for those recovering from injury, illness, or even a stroke. It indicates that progress is not lost forever. Even after prolonged inactivity, the body retains a blueprint for movement and strength. With consistency, the recovery process can access those preserved pathways to restore what was once strong.

Bottom Line: Muscle memory is genuine, enduring, and a crucial factor in accelerating recovery and enhancing performance. So, whether you're starting over or continuing your comeback, remember—your body remembers. You're not starting from scratch; you're starting from experience.

Getting Approval Before Starting Exercise: Before starting any exercise program, especially for those who are overweight or have health issues like high blood pressure, diabetes, or joint problems, it's crucial to get a doctor's approval.

> If you're 50-100 pounds overweight, you face a higher risk of injury and should proceed with caution, particularly if you have type 2 diabetes or high blood pressure. **Always consult your healthcare provider** to ensure your exercise plan is safe and suitable for your needs.

Resistance Training

1. The Role of Resistance Training: Resistance training is a crucial part of any fitness regimen, particularly as we age or if we are overweight. **It enhances bone density, builds muscle mass, and improves overall strength—essential factors for maintaining structural health and mobility over time**. More than just lifting weights, resistance training encompasses **any method that challenges the muscles against gravity, including bodyweight exercises, resistance bands, or other forms of external resistance**. By regularly participating in this type of training, we foster long-term health, functionality, and physical resilience.

Exercises like jumping jacks and arm circles qualify as calisthenics, just like push-ups and pull-ups. *However, because you're working against your body weight and gravity, the latter two exercises also fall under the category of resistance training*. Proper technique and safety are crucial for preventing injury, especially when lifting heavier weights or if you have pre-existing health conditions. *As muscle mass increases, the body burns calories more efficiently, losing fat and improving body composition.*

2. Resistance training is an essential component of a fitness plan for individuals with obesity or significant weight gain. However, it must be tailored to the individual's level of fitness and ability. It's not a one-size-fits-all approach; specific exercises may not suit everyone. For example, not everyone can perform tire flips or box jumps safely. The key is to create a workout plan tailored to your fitness level, limitations, and goals.

After a workout, your body continues to burn calories at an increased rate for 36-48 hours, a phenomenon known as "post-exercise oxygen (**EPOC**) consumption." This means that even after you've finished exercising, your body is still working to repair and rebuild muscle fibers, which burns calories. The intensity of your resistance training determines how long this increased calorie burn persists. There's a lot of hype around EPOC, and many gyms use it as a selling point. While it's real, **EPOC (Excess Post-Exercise Oxygen Consumption)** only accounts for about **6–15%** additional calorie burn post-workout, according to the **American Council on Exercise** and the *Journal of Sports Sciences*—making it a modest bonus, not a primary fat-loss tool.

3. The Importance of Technique and Proper Progression: Whether you're lifting weights or doing bodyweight exercises, technique is crucial. Poor form can lead to injuries, particularly for those who are overweight or new to resistance training. Begin with manageable weights or resistance and concentrate on mastering the form before increasing the intensity. Progress gradually to allow your body to adapt and minimize the risk of injury.

4. Building Muscle for Better Health: Building muscle mass, or rather its density, is crucial for enhancing overall body composition, particularly for individuals carrying excess weight. Increased muscle mass supports your skeletal structure, making daily activities easier and reducing strain on your joints. Stronger muscles also improve balance, posture, and metabolism, all of which are essential for long-term health and well-being.

> **Conclusion:** Resistance training is crucial for everyone, especially those who are overweight or obese, as it enhances strength, bone density, and metabolism. Exercise safely by using proper techniques and maintaining an appropriate intensity level for your fitness level. Always consult a doctor before starting a new program, particularly if you have health issues. Gradually build strength and listen to your body's limitations.

Key Concepts of TUT – Time Under Tension

TUT refers to the total duration your muscles are under strain during an exercise. By slowing down movement tempo, this method increases muscular stress, which can enhance muscle growth, strength, and endurance. TUT emphasizes slower, more controlled reps. Instead of a typical 1-second up / 1-second down tempo (1/1), TUT might involve a 3–5 second duration for each phase of movement.

- Example: Lowering the weight in 4 seconds and raising it in 3 seconds significantly increases the time the muscle is under load.

- This slower pace makes a given weight feel heavier, increasing muscle fiber recruitment and metabolic stress.

Sufficient Weight Is Crucial: To maximize the effectiveness of TUT, your working weight should be at least **60% of your one-rep max (1RM).**

- For example, if your 1RM for a bicep curl is 50 lbs, a TUT set should use at least 30 lbs.

- Using weights that are too light may not stimulate sufficient muscle growth. However, newer studies show hypertrophy can still occur with **15–20 reps using lighter weights**—though this is more common in general fitness training than in bodybuilding or advanced programs.

Muscle Activation and Growth: TUT helps activate **deeper muscle fibers** that may not be fully engaged with faster reps or heavier, shorter sets.

Progressive Overload Still Applies: Muscle adaptation still requires **progression**. If you consistently use the same weight—even with TUT—you'll likely hit a plateau. Adjust intensity, reps, or tempo to keep advancing.

Scientific Insights on TUT

- A 5-second tempo (both up and down) can increase TUT by 40%, but this may reduce the total number of reps you can or should perform.

- Faster tempos allow more overall training volume (sets × reps × weight), which contributes to hypertrophy when volume is the main focus.

- Both tempo and volume play important roles in a balanced strength program.

Benefits of TUT

- Improves muscle strength and endurance by increasing fiber and motor unit activation

- Stimulates protein synthesis—essential for muscle repair and growth

- Helps overcome plateaus by introducing new muscular challenges

- Increases **mind-muscle connection**, encouraging greater control and focus

Practical Application of TUT

- During training **plateaus**

- While transitioning to **heavier loads**

- When refining **movement control and technique**

Tempo Variations: Example — Biceps Curl

Try different cadences like:

- **3–1–2**: 3 seconds down, 1-second pause, 2 seconds up

- **3–1–2–1**: Add 1-second pause at the top

There are many other variations, but these cover most common training needs.

Combine with Other Methods

TUT complements—but does not replace other proven techniques like:

- Progressive overload

- Drop sets

- Supersets

- Traditional hypertrophy or strength cycles

Eccentric and Concentric Focus

The **eccentric phase** (lengthening of the muscle) especially benefits from TUT.

- Slowing the eccentric movement increases muscle fiber recruitment and builds structural strength.

- Legendary bodybuilder **Mike Mentzer** was known for using eccentric-focused reps—called "negatives"—in short, high-intensity sessions.

- His approach, inspired by **Dr. Arthur Jones** (inventor of Nautilus machines), emphasized **quality over quantity**. While not ideal for everyone, it proved highly effective for Mentzer and many others.

Limitations of TUT

- Leads to **faster fatigue**, potentially reducing total reps or sets

- Not suitable for **every exercise or training goal**

- Should be used to **complement**, not dominate, your training program

Final Thoughts

Time Under Tension is a powerful method to boost muscle activation, promote growth, and improve movement control. It's especially useful when you're stuck in a plateau or want to sharpen your form and intensity.

Used wisely and in balance with other training methods, TUT can add depth to your workouts, challenge your muscles in new ways, and help you reach your fitness goals more efficiently.

Changing Routines

When Change Becomes Necessary

For most people, **resistance training routines should be adjusted or changed every 4 to 8 weeks**, depending on several factors such as:

1. **Training Age (Experience Level):**

   - **Beginners:** Can stick with the same program for 8–12 weeks, since they adapt more slowly and still see gains.

   - **Intermediate to Advanced:** May benefit from changing routines every 4–6 weeks to avoid plateaus.

2. **Progress & Adaptation:**

   - If you're no longer gaining strength, size, or endurance—or feel bored or stagnant—it's time to adjust.

   - Progress can be made by increasing weight, reps, sets, intensity, or changing tempo—**not just switching exercises.**

3. **Goals:**

    ◦ If your goal shifts (e.g., from hypertrophy to fat loss or strength to endurance), your routine should change accordingly.

Ways to "Change" a Routine Without Scrapping It:

- Change rep ranges (e.g., 12–15 → 6–8)

- Switch to a new exercise variation (e.g., barbell squat → goblet squat)

- Alter your rest periods

- Shift your training split (e.g., full-body → push/pull/legs)

- Adjust tempo or use advanced methods like supersets or drop sets

Bottom Line: Change **intelligently, not constantly.** Stick with a plan long enough to make progress, but not so long that your body and mind go stale. For most people, reviewing your routine every **4–8 weeks** is a good sweet spot.

Lactate Threshold

Push Past the Burn: Understanding Your Lactate Threshold

Lactate threshold is the exercise intensity at which lactate starts to accumulate in the blood faster than the body can clear it. This marks a physiological tipping point where energy demands begin to exceed the limits of purely aerobic metabolism. As intensity increases, the body shifts toward anaerobic energy production, leading to a buildup of lactate and associated hydrogen ions.

The Science Behind It

During low-to moderate-intensity exercise, the body mainly depends on aerobic metabolism. Glucose and fatty acids are broken down in the mitochondria, generating energy efficiently with few by products. As exercise intensity increases, the body demands ATP faster than aerobic processes can provide. Anaerobic glycolysis takes over, producing

ATP quickly but less efficiently. A byproduct of this process is lactate. While lactate can be used as fuel by other tissues, the rise in hydrogen ions also contributes to muscle acidity and fatigue. At levels below the lactate threshold, the body can eliminate lactate as fast as it is produced. Above the threshold, lactate builds up, impeding muscle function. contraction and reducing performance.

How Athletes Improve It – <u>NOT</u> for beginners!

Training at or just above the lactate threshold leads to key physiological adaptations:

- **Increased mitochondrial density**: Improves the muscle's capacity for aerobic energy production.

- **Enhanced lactate clearance**: Muscles become more efficient at using lactate as fuel.

- **Improved buffering capacity**: The body better neutralizes hydrogen ions to resist pH changes.

- **Greater capillary density**: Enhances blood flow, oxygen delivery, and waste removal.

- **Upregulation of lactate transporters (MCT1 and MCT4)**: Facilitates more efficient lactate movement in and out of muscle cells.

- These adaptations allow athletes to sustain higher intensities for longer durations without fatigue caused by lactate buildup. Raising the lactate threshold is one of the most effective ways to improve endurance performance.

NEGATIVE & ISOMETRIC TRAINING

NEGATIVE movements, also known as **eccentric** movements, refer to the phase of an exercise when you're resisting the pull of gravity or the apparatus.
- During the negative phase, muscles lengthen under tension, which is highly

effective for strength and muscle development.

- Eccentric training uniquely engages muscle fibers, promoting strength and growth.

- Controlled Descent: Always release the weight (or your body) ***slowly & steadily*** during the negative phase. Avoid letting it drop, or moving too quickly.

Benefits of Negative Movements:
- Activates more muscle fibers, increasing strength.

- Creates controlled tension, which enhances muscle endurance and stability.

- Reducing the risk of injury by improving control during exercises.

Timing:
- Standard negatives: Lower for 1-2 seconds.

- Advanced negatives: 10 to 20 seconds or longer for added intensity, depending on the actual movement.

- Remember that the number of reps and sets matters significantly.

Examples of Negative Movements in Common Exercises:
- Push-ups: Lower yourself slowly, aiming for 5-20 seconds during the descent; we have gone as long as 60- 90 seconds.

- Pull-ups: Slowly lower your body for 3-5 seconds after pulling up.

- Bicep Curls: Control the lowering phase for 2-4 seconds while maintaining proper form.

Incorporating negative movements into your workouts can enhance strength and endurance, particularly during the last 1-2 sets. You can target a muscle group using these alone, but only if you are physically prepared and understand the scientific principles behind this method.

Common Mistakes to Avoid
- Dropping the Weight Too Quickly.

- Using Momentum: Avoid swinging or jerking movements to "cheat" through the exercise unless it is controlled – "**Focus on controlled motion**."

- Skipping the Negative Phase in Exercises. Ignoring a movement's eccentric (or "negative") phase—can limit muscle engagement and reduce gains. The key is control. Whether you take one second or three, always ensure that the eccentric portion of the movement is controlled. That's where a lot of growth occurs.

Advanced Negative Training:

For more experienced lifters or athletes, advanced negative training can involve:
- Extended Negatives: Lower for up to 10-30 seconds per repetition, typically used for only a few reps and sets.

- Assisted Negatives: Use a partner or machine to help with the positive phase, allowing you to focus entirely on the negative.

- Overloaded Negatives: Incorporate heavier weights during the eccentric phase with adequate support, often referred to as a forced negative move. I learned this in the **Nautilus training system**, developed by Dr. Arthur Jones, from Mr. Gary S. in 1975 who trained at the Nautilus facility in Deland, Florida, and was also involved during the time of the Colorado experiment with Casey Viator. I advise working with a highly proficient trainer in this discipline, typically only found among professional athlete coaches.

The Takeaway: Negative movements are a powerful tool to enhance your workout routine. They activate more muscle fibers, build strength, and improve control. Controlled eccentric training ensures you're maximizing your efforts in each exercise.

Incorporating negatives into your final sets is especially effective for building strength and endurance.

Remember: Concentrate on form, control, and timing during negative movements. Consult with a seasoned professional in isometric and negative movement training for any questions or guidance you may need.

Proper body mechanics should be followed—**to a point**. Not every body is built the same, and not everyone can safely perform movements according to a textbook ideal. For example, some individuals cannot squat to parallel or below parallel due to structural differences, mobility limitations, or injury history.

Because of this, proper form is **not simply a universal standard**. Proper form is what your body can perform safely and effectively. The best form for *you* is the form that does not place you at unnecessary risk while allowing the intended muscles to do the work.

If your alignment is controlled, your movement is stable, and the correct muscles are engaged without pain or strain, then your form is most likely both proper and safe.

Isometrics

Isometric exercises involve holding a position or exerting force without any noticeable movement in the joints. By maintaining tension in a fixed position, this training builds strength and engages multiple muscle fibers.

Incorporating Isometrics into Your Training - Repetitions: Perform 2-3 sets per exercise; any more is strictly not advised, with a 45-60 second rest between sets.

Types of:
- Yielding: Holding a position or object that might move slightly under tension.

- Overcoming: Pushing or pulling against an immovable object.

Benefits of Isometric Training

- Builds foundational strength.

- Activates numerous muscle fibers and neurons, improving control and endurance.

- Enhances stabilization and strength in weak ranges of motion.

- Widely used by professional athletes, powerlifters, bodybuilders, martial artists, and even NASCAR drivers.

- Common in rehabilitation therapy to regain strength after surgery or injury.

Examples of Yielding Isometrics
- Loop Band Hold: Stand on a heavy-resistance loop band, putting the band over your wrists. Hold your arms bent out at a 45-degree angle. Force upward, holding the position as hard as possible for 20-30 seconds, engaging your calves, thighs, glutes, core, and back. If you start trembling, you have the correct intensity; <u>take many small breaths and do NOT hold your breath</u>!

- Medicine Ball Squeeze: Hold a (slam ball) in front of your chest. Squeeze the ball as hard as possible, tensing your entire body for 20-30 seconds.

- Push-Up Hold: Lower yourself one-third, halfway, or three-quarters of the way down in a push-up position. Hold for 30-60 seconds, depending on your strength. You can also do so at each elevation.

- Hold a barbell straight out, engaging your core muscles 20-30 seconds; this was Bruce Lee's go to and now also mine.

Examples of Overcoming Isometrics
- In overcoming isometrics, you exert maximum force against an immovable object.

- Wall Push: Stand before a wall with your palms pressed against it, and push as hard as possible, engaging your entire body for 20-30 seconds.

- Set up inside a squat rack with the bar positioned between waist height and just below your pecs. Place a pad on the bar for comfort.

- **Push down:** Drive the edge of your palms into the bar, pressing downward with maximum force – use caution & control your breathing.

- **Push up:** Shift pressure so the bar rests just below your thumbs. Drive upward as hard as you can. To make this effective, load the bar with heavy weight or use an immovable setup such as a Smith machine locked in place use caution & control your breathing.

- The bar itself should not move. By pushing down and then up against an immovable object, you generate constant tension in both directions. This extended time under tension recruits more motor units, strengthens neural pathways, and trains your muscles to contract harder and rebuild stronger.

Special Applications of Isometric Training
Weak Point Training:
- For bench press hold the bar at the weakest point (e.g., three-quarters of the way up) for 10-20 seconds.

- **Have a spotter** for safety when working with heavy weights.

Martial Arts & Functional Strength:
- Martial artists often hold low squats or balance positions to develop incredible strength without adding bulk.

- They may also punch and block in a deliberate, <u>slow</u> move under <u>constant tension</u>.

- These positions develop static strength, which is critical for combat and balance.

Common Mistakes to Avoid
- Insufficient Effort: Not exerting maximum force defeats the purpose of isometric training.

- Poor Form: Always maintain proper posture to prevent injury and maximize results.

- The duration of an isometric hold depends on both the intensity and the type of exercise. For example, holding a push-up at one-third or two-thirds of the way down can typically be sustained for 20 to 30 seconds without risk of injury. In fact, my personal best was a 2-minute hold at one-third from the bottom.

- That said, the level of exertion matters. A push-up hold is challenging, but it's not maximal effort. It's very different from squeezing a medicine ball with all your strength or pushing against a wall or doorframe until your entire body shakes. Those types of all-out isometric efforts place significantly more strain on muscles, tendons,and ligaments, and in those cases, you must be cautious with time under tension to avoid injury.

The Takeaway

Isometric exercises effectively build strength and stability without movement. Use yielding isometrics for slight movements with sustained tension, and overcoming isometrics to exert force against immovable objects.

Incorporating these exercises into your routine can help enhance strength, address areas of weakness, and improve endurance. They are essential for athletes, bodybuilders, and martial artists looking to develop power and control.

> "FITNESS IS TO THE BODY WHAT KNOWLEDGE IS TO THE MIND"

Mind-Muscle Connection

Maximize workout effectiveness by engaging both body and mind. The **mind-muscle connection**, being aware and intentional with each movement, transforms workouts, yielding better results in less time. Here's a structured breakdown.

Practical training requires full mental engagement. Treat each rep as an opportunity to connect with the muscles you're working.

Avoid Distractions: Intense exercise limits the feasibility of long conversations. Keep communication brief and targeted between sets and concentrate fully on the exercise during each movement. Relying on subconscious familiarity with the movement isn't enough; staying present is essential.

Efficient Training Duration – Time Commitment: Research shows 45–75 minutes is the typical range for effective strength or endurance training. Most adaptations—strength, hypertrophy, and aerobic fitness—are achieved in this window if intensity and volume are appropriate, and even shorter sessions of 20–30 minutes can be effective when well-designed. Training far beyond 75 minutes can increase fatigue and elevate cortisol, though the effect depends on nutrition, recovery, and fitness level. There is no universal cut-off where hormones shift negatively, and well-conditioned athletes may train longer without harm because their recovery and fueling strategies offset the stress.

Intensity and Planning: Tailor your intensity based on the day's plan: heavy vs. light, low vs. high volume.

The Role of Mind-Muscle Awareness – Visualize the Movement: Before starting an exercise, imagine the muscles you'll engage.

Example: For pull-ups, focus on engaging your back muscles, specifically the area around your shoulder blades, to ensure proper activation rather than overusing your arms.

Engagement is Key: Contract the target muscles actively during every repetition. Proper positioning and engagement should happen ***before*** starting the movement, not just during it.

Steps to Maximize Mind-Muscle Connection: Prepare Your Body. Assume the correct training position and align your body and muscles to perform the movement effectively.

> **Visualize Muscle Activation:** Mentally connect with the muscles you'll be working; envision them contracting and controlling the motion, and then actually do it. Avoid "going through the motions." **Be intentional with every rep.** Proper technique ensures that the correct muscles are engaged and reduces the risk of injury. A strong mind-muscle connection helps target the intended muscles, improving both strength and development. Training with this level of focus creates a profound impact, enhancing the quality of your workouts while reducing wasted effort.

Practical training isn't about endless hours in the gym; it's about being present, intentional, and fully engaged. OWN YOUR SPACE! Master the mind-muscle connection to unlock real progress.

> - **Lift PURE.** *It's not about moving weight but activating muscle fibers. Stimulate, don't annihilate.* Form and precision always come first.
> - Clear out negativity before every set. Give it your all. Promise yourself you'll push beyond your limits and become your best.
> - **When you train, "own the moment."** Focus. Don't drift. Work it, kill it, change your life.

Make Each Rep Count

Change your workout effectiveness— Get 100% Out of Every Rep

1. A Lesson from My Father

Despite being an amputee, my father was a three-time AAU gold medalist on the flying rings in the 1940s, a two-time U.S. amputee golf champion, and a 13-time Southern States and 12-time Florida state amputee golf champion. He lost his leg at age 11 but maintained an impressive 76 average on the golf course.

While hitting balls at the range, he shared a crucial lesson: "Son, don't simply hit the ball to complete the bucket; imagine each shot is the winning stroke for the PGA Championship." Years later, this advice resonated with me and influenced my approach to all activities, from martial arts to fitness training.

2. Applying the Lesson to Martial Arts, calisthenics, and weightlifting

I began a dedicated fitness regimen **between the ages of nineteen and twenty-two** and progressed quickly, at times outperforming martial arts opponents ranked well above me. I was never well known; I was just an average, everyday guy who became quite skilled in these disciplines.

My approach was simple: Every punch, kick, and rep mattered.

Specifically in the martial arts; instead of mindlessly repeating movements 100, or even 500 times, I treated each strike as if it needed to deliver maximum impact. This mindset was rooted in the philosophy of Shotokan karate and the "one punch, one kill" [to end a fight] Motto. It emphasized precision, focus, and intent, where every action carried a purpose. In weight lifting, I endeavored to make every rep proper and effective.

3. Bringing Focus to Fitness Training: This mindset is crucial in fitness. Too often, people focus on simply reaching a number—like 12 reps—without truly engaging in each repetition with intention and control.

> **My approach:** Every rep should matter, don't rush just to finish a set, **make each movement deliberate and purposeful. Perform every repetition as if it were the only one, with full focus and effort**. While a single rep won't build strength on its own, how you approach each rep—the first, the second, the third—determines your progress. Treat each repetition as an opportunity to grow stronger, whether it's pull-ups, push-ups, squats, or rows. The objective is not merely to finish the set, but to intelligently challenge your limits by training with purpose.

4. The Value of Effort Over Numbers

Reaching muscle failure (exhaustion) in a set isn't a sign of weakness; it's a testament to giving your all.

For example:

- If you aim for 10 reps but can only complete 9.5 with proper form, that effort counts more than forcing the 10th with poor technique.

- **It's about maximizing each movement, not just hitting arbitrary numbers.**

- **Mindful Training: Focus on proper form, rhythm, and execution. Each rep should feel meaningful, whether it's your first or last.**

Effort is Key: Training to or near muscle failure can be essential for effectively challenging your muscles, but it doesn't need to happen in every set. The right approach depends on **your experience and ability**. For most people, reaching failure on every set is ***not*** necessary. Instead, focus on pushing yourself while maintaining good form. If you train to failure, reserve it for the last one or two reps of your final set—unless you're a highly experienced weightlifter or bodybuilder, like the late Mr. Mike Mentzer, who held the titles of: Mr. America, Mr. Universe, and Mr. Olympia.

Intentional Exercise: Whether you're a casual exerciser or a dedicated athlete, put your heart and soul into every movement.

> **Final Thought:** Making every rep count is a mindset that goes beyond fitness. It's about being present, giving your best effort, and treating every action as if it truly matters. Whether in the gym or in life, this approach can lead to remarkable growth and success.

The Myth Of Muscle Confusion

The notion of "muscle confusion," a popularized fitness concept, is fundamentally flawed. Contrary to this misleading term, muscles do not possess the cognitive capacity to become "confused." The actual mechanism behind the effectiveness of varying exercises lies in the targeted stimulation of different muscle fibers and regions within the same muscle group.

For instance, while both hammer curls and regular curls engage the biceps, they emphasize different aspects of the muscle. Hammer curls, with their neutral grip, primarily target the brachialis, a muscle located beneath the biceps, and engage the forearm more, while regular curls place greater emphasis on the biceps brachii itself.

Experienced athletes and bodybuilders, recognizing the limitations of the "confusion" theory, adhere to a structured training regimen. They understand that real progress comes from a focused approach that emphasizes important elements, including intensity, frequency, and specific muscle groups in their workouts.

When to Shake Things Up: Recognizing the Need for Change

The primary reasons for introducing changes to your workout regimen are based on practical considerations, not the mythical concept of "muscle confusion."

Combat Boredom: Stagnation can quickly set in if your workouts become monotonous. Introducing new exercises, exploring different training modalities, or simply rearranging your routine can combat boredom and reignite your motivation.

Breaking Through Plateaus: When progress stalls, it's crucial to analyze your training approach.

- **Are you pushing yourself to your limits?** Are you consistently challenging yourself to lift heavier weights, perform more repetitions, or hold isometric contractions for longer durations?

- **Are you adequately balancing training intensity?** For optimal results, it is crucial to incorporate a mix of heavy lifting days, focusing on strength and power, with lighter days that emphasize higher repetitions and muscular endurance, particularly for experienced individuals.

- **Are you training all major muscle groups?** A well-rounded training program should address all major muscle groups, ensuring balanced development and minimizing the risk of imbalances.

- **Are you consistently challenging your body?** The principle of progressive overload is paramount for continued growth. This involves gradually increasing the demands placed on your body, whether through incremental increases in weight, repetitions, or the introduction of more challenging variations of exercises.

Progressive Training: A Cornerstone of Strength Gains

Progressive training is a systematic and highly effective approach to achieving consistent gains. It involves a gradual and methodical increase in training intensity over time. This can be achieved through various means:

- **Increasing the load:** Gradually adding weight to the bar or increasing the resistance bands.

- **Increasing the volume:** Performing more repetitions or sets of a given exercise.

- **Increasing resistance:** Using tools like weight vests, resistance bands, or chains can enhance resistance in workouts. Powerlifters exemplify progressive overload by focusing on heavy, low-repetition lifts such as deadlifts and squats, prioritizing strength and ample recovery. Their success highlights the benefits of gradually increasing weight over time.

The Importance of Recognizing When Change is Unnecessary

Recognize that change isn't always necessary. If you're satisfied with your fitness progress, don't disrupt your routine. However, when you hit plateaus or desire a new challenge, it's time to reevaluate your training strategy.

Chapter 6
STRENGTH TRAINING FOR FAT LOSS MATTERS

One of the most debated topics in fitness is whether cardio or strength training is more effective for fat loss. Cardio makes you sweat, burns calories fast, and feels productive—but when it comes to long-term fat loss, preserving lean muscle, and keeping your metabolism running strong, strength training comes out ahead.

The Problem With Cardio-Only Weight Loss

Relying solely on cardio often leads to initial weight loss—**but not the right kind**. Without resistance training, much of that weight comes from muscle. That's a problem, because muscle is what keeps your metabolism humming.

When muscle is lost:

- Your resting metabolic rate drops.

- You burn fewer calories at rest.

- You become more prone to weight regain and energy crashes.

> Cardio also trains the body for **efficiency**, not fat-burning. Over time, your body learns to burn fewer calories to do the same work. That means unless you keep increasing cardio or slashing calories, results stall.

What Cardio Signals to the Body

Cardio's main adaptation is endurance—not muscle growth. Your body responds by:
- **Reducing muscle mass** to conserve energy

- Becoming more **efficient** (fewer calories burned at rest)

- Increasing cravings and hunger due to **hormonal shifts**

While some cardio has its place, overemphasis can create a "skinny fat" appearance—lower body weight, but low muscle tone and a sluggish metabolism.

Why Strength Training Wins

Strength training sends a different message: **"We need to be strong."** This stimulus helps preserve and build muscle even in a calorie deficit. It promotes:
- **Muscle retention and growth**

- **Increased calorie burn at rest** (through EPOC and lean mass)

- **Hormonal balance** that supports sustainable fat loss

- **You don't just lose weight—you reshape your body and rev up your metabolism.**

Combine Both (But Smartly)

You don't need to ditch cardio altogether. Instead:
- Prioritize strength training 3x/week with compound lifts

- Add cardio 2–3x/week, ideally after weights or on separate days

- Use circuits or supersets if you're short on time

> For Fat Loss, Start With Muscle and Let Cardio Support—Not Sabotage—Your Results.

To Avoid Burnout and Metabolic Slowdown:
- Create a **modest calorie deficit** (300–500/day) – see a nutritionist!

- **Eat enough protein** to preserve lean mass

- **Train consistently**, but don't overdo it

- Allow for **gradual, sustainable progress**

Crash diets and endless cardio might work short-term, but they set you up for long-term setbacks. Muscle is your metabolic armor—build it, and you'll burn fat smarter, not harder.

Not All Weight Training Is Equal

Lifting weights is not just about time under the bar—it's about the method, intensity, and structure. Many people assume 45 minutes of lifting is enough, but without the right approach, those minutes may not yield real progress. The effectiveness of resistance training depends on how you train, not just how long you train.

There are different styles of weight training that serve different goals:
- **Powerlifters** focus on maximum strength, using heavy weights and low reps in core lifts such as the squat, deadlift, and bench press.

- **Bodybuilders** aim for hypertrophy, building muscle size with moderate to heavy weights and higher training volume.

- **Recreational lifters or group class participants** often use very light dumbbells (e.g., 5 lbs) in circuit formats or high-rep workouts. These raise the heart rate and improve endurance but provide limited stimulus for muscle growth.

- *Extremely light weights that never bring the muscle near fatigue do not create the micro-tears in muscle fibers that drive repair, growth, and metabolic improvement.*

What About HIIT with Weights?

High-Intensity Interval Training (HIIT) with weights combines resistance and cardio for a fast-paced, fat-burning approach. **It can be very effective—if the weights are meaningful.**

If you're using very light dumbbells and performing high reps without fatigue, you're doing more cardio than resistance training. True body transformation comes from muscular challenge, not just movement.

Bottom line: HIIT with weights works only if the loads are heavy enough to engage your muscles. Otherwise, you're just exercising—not strength training.

The Goal for Fat Loss: **Build Lean Muscle Density, Not Bulk, (unless you want to)** — Muscle is metabolically active tissue. The more muscle you carry, the more calories you burn at rest.

DON'T BURN OFF THE FAT, WORK IT OFF

Building lean muscle:
- Raises your resting metabolic rate (RMR)

- Increases fat-burning efficiency

- Helps recompose and reshape your body without adding unwanted size.

You don't need to "bulk up" to see results. You need to build muscle that helps you burn calories even when you're not at the gym.

The Foundation: Compound Movements

The fastest path to strength and fat loss is through compound exercises—multi-joint movements that work several muscle groups at once.

Examples include:
- Squats
- Deadlifts
- Bench Press
- Overhead Press
- Rows
- Pull-Ups

These lifts recruit more muscle, increase hormonal response (like testosterone and growth hormone), and create the micro-damage that drives muscular repair and metabolic change.

Isolation Exercises: Use Them Later

Isolation exercises like curls or leg extensions target one muscle at a time. They can be great for shaping and definition, but they shouldn't be your priority in a fat-loss phase. Use isolation work to refine your body after the foundation is built through compound lifts.

Cardio Alone Isn't Enough

Many people rely on cardio for fat loss. But done excessively, especially in a calorie deficit, it can backfire.

Potential issues with too much steady-state cardio:

- Metabolic slowdown

- Muscle loss

- Hormonal disruptions (like elevated cortisol, which increases fat storage)

Cardio has its place—but resistance training is what protects your muscle and keeps your metabolism strong.

Sprinters vs. Long-Distance Runners: A Contrast

Sprinters train with short, explosive movements. They build muscle, power, and rely on fast-twitch fibers.

Distance runners train with low-intensity, long-duration activity. They build endurance but often lose muscle mass, relying more on slow-twitch fibers with lower muscle density.

The contrast is easy to see—and it reflects the way each athlete trains

Best Strategy for Fat Loss and Muscle Retention

- Strength train 3–4 days per week

- Add moderate cardio (such as HIIT or walking) a few times weekly

- Prioritize protein intake

- Avoid severe calorie restriction

- Use progressive overload (increase resistance or challenge gradually)

To Make Strength Training Effective

- Use weights that challenge you. The last few reps should feel difficult, but doable with good form.

- Avoid extremely high reps with light weights unless you're doing it for endurance specifically.

- Workouts can be 30–45+ minutes long.

- Adjust rest periods to match your goal:
  - Muscle endurance: 20–90 seconds rest
  - Strength/hypertrophy: 2–3 minutes rest

High-Intensity Training Tips

HIIT and circuit workouts are time-efficient and metabolically powerful. Add explosive moves like:

- Kettlebell swings
- Plyometric jumps
- Medicine ball slams
- Sled pushes or battle ropes

These build power while burning fat rapidly.

Time and Intensity: What's Enough?

Fat loss doesn't require hours in the gym. Consistency and effort matter more.

Aim for:

- 150 minutes of moderate to intense training **per week**
- 3 to 4 sessions weekly lasting 30–45 minutes

- Sessions that challenge you, not exhaust you

"Moderate" doesn't mean easy—it means sustainable and effective.

Final Fat Loss Tips

- Focus on consistency, not perfection
- Increase weights or intensity over time
- Prioritize form and recovery
- Choose the right program for your age, ability, and schedule
- Progress slowly, and celebrate steady gains

> **Key Takeaway:** Cardio burns calories. Strength training drives body recomposition—reducing fat, building lean muscle, and raising metabolism. Train smart, train with purpose, and stay consistent. The goal is a leaner, stronger, healthier you—not just during your workout, but all day long.

Why The Scale Goes Up Before It Goes Down

It's common to experience slight weight gain in the first few weeks of starting a fitness program, especially one that involves resistance training. This temporary gain is not a sign of failure but rather part of your body's natural adaptation process.

Micro-Trauma and Inflammation:

- Resistance training causes tiny tears in muscle fibers (micro-trauma).
- Your body initiates a healing process that results in temporary inflammation.
- To repair the muscle, your body retains fluid around the damaged areas, leading to water weight gain.

Increased Glycogen Storage:

- When you exercise regularly, your body stores more glycogen to fuel your workouts.

- Glycogen binds with water in a 1:3 ratio (1 gram of glycogen binds with 3 grams of water). This combination adds weight, but it's a healthy and necessary process to improve energy levels for exercise.

Delayed-Onset Muscle Soreness (DOMS)
- DOMS occurs 1-2 days after a workout and is a natural response to the micro-tears in muscle tissue.

- This soreness is a sign that your muscles are adapting to the new stress and building strength.

Why These Changes Are Temporary
- Water Retention Reduces Over Time

- As your muscles adapt to exercise, they experience less micro-trauma and inflammation.

- Your body retains less fluid, and water weight begins to drop.

Efficiency in Energy Usage:
- Initially, your muscles store more glycogen to fuel exercise.

- Over time, as your body becomes more efficient, it requires less glycogen to maintain the same energy output.

- This reduction in glycogen storage means less water is bound to your muscles, leading to weight stabilization or loss.

- Expect an initial fluctuation in weight (1-5 pounds, depending on body size).

- After a few weeks, water retention decreases, and muscle efficiency improves.

- With consistent effort in exercise and proper nutrition, weight loss and body composition changes will follow.

Important Tips for Managing Expectations

- Don't Panic: Weight gain initially is temporary, not fat gain.

- **Track Progress Beyond the Scale:** Use measurements, photos, or <u>how clothes fit to monitor progress</u>.

Carbohydrates and Recovery: Avoid restricting carbs completely (unless on a specific *short-term* low carb diet recommended by a qualified Nutritionist), as they're essential for replenishing glycogen stores. You can consume healthy carbs after workouts to support recovery and energy levels.

Key Takeaway: When starting a fitness program, initial weight gain is normal and results from inflammation and glycogen storage. As you train consistently, your body will adapt, leading to fat loss and improved fitness. Trust the process!

The Scale:

The scale's usefulness varies. Regular weigh-ins help some stay motivated—79% of successful weight losers tracked weekly—but for others, it can overshadow progress. Weight loss isn't linear; daily fluctuations of 3–5 lbs. are normal due to hydration, food, and exercise. Muscle gain from strength training can at times, mask fat loss.

The scale reflects a moment, not trends. **Hormonal changes and muscle gain can affect weight. So instead, track body measurements, clothing fit, and fitness progress for a complete picture.** Weight isn't the only indicator of health. *Improvements in energy levels, mood, sleep quality, and overall well-being are important outcomes that the scale cannot measure.*

A Slip Is Not All That Unusual:

A slip isn't failure. Don't let guilt lead to more splurging—treat it as a learning moment. Even trainers indulge, and one cheat meal won't derail progress. If resisting is hard, plan a cheat every 3–4 weeks and focus on better strategies next time.

Poor Diet: Both overeating and undereating can hinder weight loss. Overeating causes fat accumulation, while *severe calorie restriction* slows metabolism and triggers survival responses, complicating weight loss. Avoid fad diets that lack essential nutrients; instead, focus on balanced meals with fruits, vegetables, whole grains, and proper portions.

Roadblocks to Weight Loss

Tracking your intake can help, and it's important not to dip too low: women should *generally* consume at least 1,200–1,500 calories daily, and men at least 1,500. Eating too little signals deprivation, causing your body to conserve energy instead of burning fat.

Insufficient Exercise: Short, low-intensity workouts won't significantly raise your heart rate or support meaningful weight loss. Infrequent moderate or intense sessions also fall short when it comes to balancing excess calorie intake. Aim for 45–60 minutes of moderate-intensity aerobic exercise, or a combination of cardio and resistance, such as *properly* designed HIIT or circuit training, designed to challenge both your heart and major muscle groups. Also, try activities like walking, running, or dancing a few days a week. **Avoid exercises targeting just one body area.**

Self-Sabotage: Unnoticed habits can stall progress. Small habits, even with good intentions, can undermine weight loss. Bingeing on sweets during cheat days is misleading. It is a "cheat meal"...mindless snacking adds up. Hidden calories in drinks like soda can easily hinder progress—one soda daily adds about 150 calories. Be mindful of your consumption, especially during screen time or social events.

Other Factors: A good weight-loss plan may face unexpected challenges that hinder calorie burning. Stress and sleep deprivation disrupt hormonal balance, impacting metabolism and increasing cravings for comfort food. Conditions like menopause, thyroid issues, or certain medications can also lead to weight gain. However, your weight might be suitable for your height and body type. If you're exercising and eating well but not losing weight, consider consulting your family physician, or an endocrinologist for an evaluation and personal recommendations.

And remember—**not everyone is meant to have the same weight or body type.** We each possess unique physiques—ectomorph, mesomorph, and endomorph. Genetics play a major role, with parents, ancestry, and heritage shaping body composition (*Heritability of BMI, NCBI; Genetic studies on body fat distribution, PMC*). **People worldwide are naturally tall, broad, or solid, while others are smaller in stature.** That's normal. Therefore, when charts or medical offices suggest that someone of a certain height and age should weigh a specific amount, that's not always accurate—or fair.

In my 50 years of fitness, I've repeatedly preached this truth: just because two people are the same age and height doesn't mean they should weigh the same. We were all made differently. God designed our bodies uniquely, and that's something to respect, not resist.

Chapter 7
HIGHLY EFFECTIVE EXERCISE METHODOLOGIES

The Best Go-To's

Walking

Walking at a slow, steady pace primarily taps into fat stores for energy, making it ideal for **reducing adipose tissue** without stressing the joints. It improves metabolic function, supports cardiovascular health, and helps regulate insulin—**while burning fat more efficiently than high-impact workouts for many.**

Aim for **30 to 60 minutes of brisk walking, 5 to 6 days a week.** Even **20-minute sessions** have benefits, especially when done consistently. For fat loss, total time matters more than speed—just keep the pace steady enough to slightly raise your heart rate while still being able to hold a conversation.

Cycling

Cycling effectively curbs appetite, burns calories, boosts metabolism, and preserves lean muscle. Interval cycling—specifically 4-minute bursts at 90% effort followed by 2-minute rests—can increase weight loss by up to 36% and improve cardiovascular fitness by approximately 13%, according to recent studies in the *Journal of Applied Physiology*.

Swimming

Swimming is a full-body, low-impact workout that burns significant calories while reducing stress on joints. A 160-pound individual can burn approximately 500 calories by swimming for one hour at a moderate pace, based on data from Harvard Medical School.

Combination Workouts

Combination workouts integrate strength, cardio, and flexibility. Forms like power yoga, hot yoga, and Bikram yoga engage nearly every muscle group. Boot camp and circuit training alternate between calisthenics (burpees, push-ups, jumping jacks) and strength components (dumbbells, weight plates) under the guidance of a personal trainer.

Calorie Burn Enhancers

Step 1: Add Weights

Adding weights increases the intensity of many aerobic exercises. For example, step aerobics burns about 347 calories in 30 minutes. Using ankle weights can raise that to nearly 500 calories. Although running with weights may increase injury risk, exercises such as rowing, stepping, and floor aerobics can be safely intensified with ankle or wrist weights.

Step 2: Use Gym Machines

Calorie burn depends on weight, intensity, and fitness level. Gym machines can provide steady effort, but numbers vary.

Running at 8 mph (treadmill, 30 min): ~372 kcal (155 lb), ~444 kcal (185 lb); heavier weights can exceed 600 kcal.

Stair stepper (30 min): ~216 kcal (155 lb), ~258 kcal (185 lb); higher body weight or faster pace can approach 400 kcal.

Low-impact aerobics (30 min): ~176 kcal (155 lb), ~204 kcal (180 lb), ~232 kcal (205 lb).

Cardio Guidelines

What Is Cardio: Cardiovascular exercise continuously engages large muscle groups (e.g., legs), increasing heart rate and respiration. Examples include walking, swimming, cycling, and skating.

Recommended Duration

- **Mayo Clinic**: At least 30 minutes of cardio on most days

- **American College of Sports Medicine (ACSM)**: 30 minutes, five days a week

Sessions can be broken into shorter segments (minimum of 10 minutes) and still provide substantial health benefits. Longer sessions burn more calories and improve fat metabolism over time.

Fueling For Fitness

Caloric Balance and Energy Storage: The body relies on calories for all functions, drawing primarily from blood glucose for immediate energy. Excess glucose is stored as glycogen in the muscles and liver. Once glycogen stores are saturated, the remaining glucose is converted into triglycerides and stored in fat cells throughout the body.

Energy Use During Exercise: As exercise begins, blood glucose levels drop, prompting the body to tap into stored glycogen and fat for fuel. Glycogen is the preferred source due to its efficient use of oxygen, especially during high-intensity activity. During low-to-moderate intensity cardio, the body shifts toward fat metabolism. For example, a 191-pound individual might burn approximately 121 calories from fat and 89 from carbohydrates during 30 minutes of lower-intensity cardio. At higher intensities, total calorie expenditure increases, drawing more heavily on both glycogen and fat reserves.

Consistent cardio leads to:

- Improved heart and lung function

- Increased capillary density

- More mitochondria in muscle cells

- Higher fat-burning enzyme levels

- Elevated regulatory proteins for endurance

Fast-Twitch Muscle Training

Understanding Muscle Fibers: You cannot change the number of these fibers, but you can enhance their performance through specific training methods.

- **Fast-twitch fibers**: Support quick, explosive movements; rely on anaerobic energy

- **Slow-twitch fibers**: Endurance-oriented; utilize oxygen efficiently

You cannot change the number of these fibers, but you can enhance their performance through specific training methods.

Sports Requiring Fast-Twitch Fibers: Football, basketball, volleyball, and tennis rely heavily on fast-twitch muscles. These muscles produce force quickly and fatigue faster than slow-twitch fibers. Oxygen intake after intense bursts is critical for recovery.

Explosive Power & Reactive Training

These workouts improve coordination, neuromuscular efficiency, and elasticity. Key examples:

- Reactive squats: Use 50% or less of your max squat weight; explode upward from halfway down

- Depth jumps: Step off a box (18–30 inches), land, and instantly rebound into a jump

- Additional drills: Sprinting, bounding, high-knee skips

Recommended volume: 3–5 reps per set, 3 sets per workout. Focus on maximal effort and clean form.

Overspeed Workouts

Overspeed training means going beyond your usual limits—running faster or farther than your target distance. That might include downhill sprints, band-assisted runs, or stretching your mileage. If you're training for a 5K, aim for 6 or 7K. For a half marathon, try going a few miles beyond. Mark Spitz, who won seven Olympic golds in 1972, trained this way under Coach Doc Counsilman. Rather than just practicing race-length swims, Doc had him go beyond to build stamina, resilience, and a deep mental edge—and it paid off.

Interval & Circuit Training

Interval Training
Alternates high-intensity work with recovery.
Example: Run 2 minutes at brisk pace, walk 2 minutes. Repeat 6–8 times.

Circuit Training
Moves through 4–10 stations of strength and cardio with short rests. Keeps heart rate elevated.
Example: Squats, push-ups, rowing machine, planks, jump rope — 45 seconds each, minimal rest.

Continuous Training
Sustains moderate effort (50–85% max) for 20–60 minutes. Improves cardiovascular fitness and endurance.
Example: 40-minute brisk walk or steady cycling.

Cross-Training
Mixes activities to prevent overuse and keep training engaging.
Example: 10 minutes jogging, 10 minutes cycling, 10 minutes elliptical.

Exercising With A Bad Back

Working out with back pain or a spinal condition requires caution, proper guidance, and realistic expectations. While staying active is essential for long-term health, not all exercises are safe for individuals with back issues. Here's how to train intelligently while protecting your spine.

Step 1: Understand Your Back Condition

Before starting or modifying your workout routine, it's critical to understand the **nature and severity of your back issue**. Ask yourself:
- Is this a temporary sore back from overuse or poor posture?
- Is it a herniated or ruptured disc?
- Has surgery been recommended or performed?

Only a qualified healthcare provider can properly diagnose your condition and help determine which exercises are safe—and which should be avoided.

Step 2: General Guidelines for Training with a Bad Back

Avoid Hyperextension or Excessive Arching

Movements that place unnecessary stress on the spine can aggravate your condition. This includes:
- Overhead presses that force your back to arch
- Back extensions without support or control
- High-impact, jarring movements

If you do perform overhead presses, keep the dumbbells aligned with your body and avoid extending past a natural range of motion.

Focus on Controlled Movements

Back-friendly training means choosing exercises that **minimize spinal compression** and allow for stable, supported posture.
- Use machines with back support when possible
- Maintain a neutral spine
- **Contract your abs to reduce strain on the lower back**

Don't Chase the Sweat

A common misconception is that sweating equals workout effectiveness. That's not true—especially when managing back pain.
- Fat loss comes from consistent, intense efforts (weight training, cardio, intervals), not just how much you sweat
- Prioritize **form, control, and recovery**
- Focus on **progressive overload** over time rather than chasing exhaustion

Final Thoughts

A back injury doesn't mean the end of your training—it means it's time to train smarter. With proper guidance, a tailored routine, and careful execution, you can stay active, reduce pain, and even build strength safely.

> ***Disclaimer:*** **I am not a medical professional. The information shared here is based on over 50 years of exercise experience. Always consult a doctor or licensed healthcare provider to assess your individual condition before starting or changing any fitness program.**

Chapter 8
BREATH CONTROL = BETTER PERFORMANCE

For Resistance & High-Intensity Exercises

- Maintain stamina.

- Reduce exhaustion.

- Perform exercises more efficiently.

- Improve recovery between exertions.

- **Power Breathing:** The act of forcefully **exhaling during the most difficult part of a lift**. This technique increases intra-abdominal pressure, stabilizing the spine and activating core muscles, which in turn improves strength, control, and safety during heavy lifts.

Basic Breathing Principles

To get started, follow these foundational rules:
- **Nose and Mouth Breathing**: Use both your nose and mouth to maximize oxygen intake and maintain a steady airflow.

- **Exhale on Exertion**: When lifting weights or performing a movement like picking up a box, inhale before the lift and **exhale at the point of exertion** (e.g., as you lift or push). One way to think is breathe out like a kiai (karate) yell at the instant of the execution of the punch/rep; but without the shrieking.

Adjusting Breathing for Resistance Training, high-intensity interval training (HIIT) or other demanding activities, **standard one-in/one-out breathing often isn't enough.** Here's how to adjust, **when you start getting exhausted:**

Breathe In and Out Rhythmically

Start with a simple pattern of one breath in and one breath out. As you begin to tire, shift to two or three short, quick inhales followed by one or two quick controlled exhales. This helps bring in more oxygen with less effort and keeps your breathing paced and efficient.

- Inhale, exhale, inhale, exhale.

- Shift to inhale-inhale, exhale (or inhale-inhale, exhale-exhale, etc.) as exhaustion sets in.

- Once you do this continuously and get the feel of the rhythm, you will see your ability not to exhaust as quickly, allowing you to go faster and further. It works!!!

- **Deep Recovery Breaths:** Periodically, take a full deep breath to fill your lungs completely, then exhale fully. This helps expand lung capacity and reset your breathing rhythm.

Running, or Walking

Use a steady in-and-out rhythm that matches your pace. For example, inhale for two steps and exhale for two. But once you start getting exhausted, shift to the short, rhythmic, quicker breaths (e.g., two in, one out) as defined above.

> Periodically, take in a DEEP breath – your lungs don't actively pull in air—they're not muscles. Instead, muscles like the diaphragm and intercostals expand your ribcage, and the lungs fill as a result."

Explanation:
- **Lungs** are **not muscles**; they cannot contract or expand on their own.

- **The diaphragm** (a dome-shaped muscle below the lungs) and **intercostal muscles** (between the ribs) contract to **expand the chest cavity**.

- This expansion **lowers the pressure inside the lungs**, causing air to **flow in** naturally (inhalation) due to the pressure difference.

Why This Method Works

Practicing proper breathing techniques offers these benefits:
- It improves oxygen delivery to muscles, reducing fatigue.

- Allows better control of heart rate during exertion.

- Increases lung capacity over time with consistent deep-breathing practice.

Real-Life Example:

A trainee performing high-intensity medicine ball slams found the exercise particularly exhausting. He immediately noticed improved stamina and recovery between sets by adjusting to rhythmic breathing and incorporating periodic deep breaths, which I have seen countless times. I used a simular approach with a half-marathoner, med-ball slams with frog hops, *plus* box jump **while perfecting rythmic breathing**, and in less than six months, she shaved 11.5 min. off her race time.

Perfect Practice Makes Perfect:

Breathing effectively requires practice, but it's worth the effort. Focus on your breathing during daily activities, such as walking, and gradually progress to more complex movements. As you refine this skill, you'll notice significant improvements in your endurance and performance. When practiced correctly, I promise you will see a big difference.

Quick Recap
- Breathe through both your nose and mouth or separately as your body needs.

- Exhale during exertion.

- Use rhythmic breathing (e.g., two breaths in, one out) when fatigued.

- Incorporate deep recovery breathing periodically.

- Be conscious of your breathing during all types of exercise.

> **With consistent practice, these techniques will help you in any physical activity, whether running, martial arts, weightlifting, HIIT, etc. Practice, adapt, and let your breathing work for you!**

Chapter 9
WALKING & CHI RUNNING

Walk For Fat Loss and Function

Walking is simple—but don't underestimate it. Done right, it's a fat-burning, stress-killing, metabolism-boosting powerhouse.

Although many sources still cite 8,000–12,000 steps per day as a fitness benchmark, recent science shows this range isn't strictly evidence-based. A July 2025 meta-analysis published in *The Lancet Public Health*, covering over 160,000 adults worldwide, found that taking approximately 7,000 steps per day yields significant health benefits—including a 47% reduction in all-cause mortality, 25% lower cardiovascular disease risk, and major reductions in cancer, diabetes, dementia, depression, and fall risk. *Beyond 7,000 steps, gains begin to plateau, meaning most individuals don't need to reach 10,000 or more to experience substantial improvements in health (Ding et al., 2025).*

Even small increases matter. Moving from a sedentary level—such as 2,000 steps—to just 4,000 steps per day offers measurable improvements in longevity and disease risk. Studies show that each additional 1,000 daily steps is associated with a 10–15% drop in cardiovascular and all-cause mortality rates. *Moderate goals such as 5,000 to 7,000 daily steps are realistic, sustainable, and more personalized than universal targets, particularly for women over 50 or those with limited mobility (Verywell Health, 2025; Science News, 2025).*

> Current expert recommendations emphasize movement consistency over arbitrary numbers. Factors such as age, baseline health, walking pace, and daily habits all influence what's "optimal" for a given individual. What matters most is regular,

> intentional movement—especially when paired with resistance training, balance work, and adequate recovery. *While higher step counts can provide additional benefits for already active individuals, the evidence confirms that consistent, moderate walking still delivers powerful results (Self Magazine, 2025).*

- Burns Calories – No joint pain, no excuses.

- Kills Stress – Less cortisol = less belly fat.

- More daily movement = more fat burn.

- Improves Insulin Sensitivity – Especially if you walk after you eat.

How To Do It
- Post-Meal Walks: 10–15 min after every meal.

- Inclines: Treadmill or hills—burn more.

- Fasted Walks: Optional. Not magic. Just walk.

- Speed & Frequency Matter

- Brisk pace = 2.5–3 mph.

- Slow strolls (<1 mph)? Not enough.

- Move every 30 minutes—2–3 min is all it takes to reset blood sugar, boost energy, and keep your metabolism lit.

Interval Walking = Next Level

- Fartlek (Sweden): Pick a landmark—walk hard to it. Recover. Repeat.

- Japanese Study: 3 min fast, 3 min slow = better fat loss, lower BP, more stamina.

- It works because you're constantly challenging your body—not just coasting.

Want to lose fat faster?
- Lift weights 3–4x/week.
- Eat in a *controlled* deficit.
- Prioritize protein, sleep, and stress management.

Walking is your base. Strength and nutrition push it into overdrive.

Daily Life Hacks
- Take the stairs.
- Park farther away.
- Move often.
- If sitting at work all day, get up every hour and walk briskly 5+ min.

Why This Works

Centenarians do it daily. They walk, move, live longer—and so will you.
No gym required. Just **walk with purpose** and do it often.

Yes—**ChiRunning** (pronounced "chee running") is a running technique that blends **Tai Chi principles** with **running form** to reduce injury and improve efficiency. It was developed by **Danny Dreyer**, a long-distance runner and Tai Chi practitioner.

Core Concepts of Chi Running

- Relaxation: Use less muscular effort; focus on loosening joints and staying light on your feet.
- Core Engagement: **Power comes from the core (not legs); think of your legs**

as wheels rather than engines.

- Midfoot Strike: Land under your center of mass to avoid overstriding.

- Cadence and Flow: Emphasizes a consistent, smooth rhythm—usually around 170–180 steps per minute.

Benefits:

- Reduces common injuries like runner's knee, shin splints, and IT band syndrome.

- Makes running more energy-efficient, especially for distance runners.

- Encourages mindfulness and body awareness while running.

Chapter 10
AB EXERCISES. BELLY FAT. SWEAT IT OFF?

Abdominal Exercises

ABS Are Made in the Gym, Revealed in the Kitchen

- Adjust reps and sets according to your fitness level.

- Perform each workout with good form and controlled movement.

- Focus on controlled breathing and core engagement.

The following target different areas based on your fitness level and goals. Some Abdominal exercises are effective, while others can strain your lower back. Instead of listing 20 or 30 exercises, I'll highlight a few that nearly anyone can do and that have proven effective for me and all my clients for many years. Proper execution is crucial, as many people perform exercises incorrectly by not engaging the intended muscles.

I will explain these and their correct techniques. Always be cautious of your lower back; seemingly simple exercises can still cause pain. In my experience, these exercises have helped those with back issues and were manageable for them.

When performed correctly a few days a week or even daily, these can increase your abdominal strength.

Crunches – A better way:

This technique can be easy on the lower back when appropriately done: Lie flat on your back, knees bent, feet flat, and direct your hands upward at a 45° angle or straight up toward the ceiling. Your goal is to **rock onto your glutes each repetition**. Each time you perform a rep, try to lift higher each time even though that is impossible; however, you will achieve full contraction every single rep.

Go easy at first. *Be sure to warm up your lower back.* Start with 10 repetitions and later build up to 15 to 25 for 2-3 sets, resting about 20 to 30 seconds between sets. **Abdominals are not about high reps; It is all about intensity.**

Leg Lifts Done Correctly:

You will not be able to do as many repetitions as the norm because *you're not focusing on your hip flexors*; instead, you're focusing mostly on your abdominals.

Lie flat on your back with your hands under your glutes, palms facing down, which elevates your glutes slightly to align your lower back.

Lie on your back with your legs extended and feet hovering about 8–10 inches off the ground. From this starting position, contract your abs tightly, allowing your shoulders to lift slightly off the floor—not by pulling with your neck, but by **initiating the movement from your abdominals**. At the same time, raise your legs another 8–10 inches in a smooth, controlled engaging motion.

The goal is not to swing or use momentum, and especially not to let your hip flexors take over. Think of your body forming a "canoe" shape—shoulders and legs rising together through abdominal contraction, holding tension through the entire movement engaging hard at the top of the leg-lift. This creates a strong isometric effect in the core.

Start with 10–15 reps for 2-3 sets, resting 20–30 seconds between sets. As with all effective ab work, it's not about how many reps you do—it's about how hard the muscle contracts.

Two Great Oblique Exercises:

1. Russian Twist

Sit on the floor with knees bent, heels resting lightly on the ground.

Lean back slightly so your torso and thighs form a "V" shape, chest up.

Hold a weight, ball, or clasp your hands in front of you.

Rotate your torso right and left in a controlled motion.

Key Point: Brace your abdominals as if preparing for a punch on every twist. This protects the lower back and ensures the obliques are doing the work.

Avoid collapsing or twisting through the lumbar spine. Move slowly, with abdominal contraction leading each turn.

2. Standing Cable (or Band) Woodchop

Anchor a cable or resistance band at shoulder height.

Stand sideways to the anchor, feet shoulder-width apart.

Hold the handle with both hands, arms extended.

Rotate your torso diagonally across your body, pulling the handle from high to low (like chopping wood).

Key Point: Keep your core braced and hips stable. Movement comes from controlled rotation, not from swinging arms or twisting the lower back.

Understanding Abdominal Muscles:

Everyone has ABS: Abdominal muscles exist beneath the fat layer. Their visibility depends on muscle development and body fat levels.

Resistance training for the abs can increase muscle thickness (hypertrophy), which makes them more visible. Training goals determine the outcome:

- **Hypertrophy-Focused (Aesthetic):** Designed to increase size and definition of the rectus abdominis.
  Example: Weighted cable crunches or decline sit-ups with added load.

- **Athletic-Focused (Functional):** Built around stability, endurance, and neuromuscular coordination to improve performance, not just appearance.
  Example: Ab wheel rollouts — challenging the core to resist extension while maintaining control and protecting the spine.

Body Fat Percentage - Visible ABS requires a low body fat percentage:

- Men: 6–15%

- Women: 14–24%

Diet is Key:
- Reducing body fat relies heavily on a calorie-controlled diet, not just exercise.

- A thousand sit-ups daily won't reveal ABS.

- *"Six-Pack in 30 Days" Claims:* These promises are misleading. Sustainable progress takes consistent effort over months, not weeks.

- The only "magic pill" is consistency: train effectively, maintain proper nutrition, and give it time.

The most critical factor in *revealing* abdominal muscles:
- Reduce calorie intake to create a calorie deficit.

- Focus on whole, nutrient-dense foods: lean protein, vegetables, healthy fats, and complex carbohydrates.

- Avoid fad diets and aim for sustainable eating habits.

Strengthen and define your abs with **controlled** exercises such as hanging knee raises with a dumbbell between your feet, kneeling cable crunches, and decline sit-ups. Focus on **slow, intentional movements with full abdominal contraction**. Whenever possible, add resistance, and avoid rushing—**feel every rep.** There are countless ways to train your abdominals, the variety is immense, but the principle remains the same: **train with intent, not just repetition.** No matter which abdominal movement you choose, **your results will depend on one key habit—conscious contraction. You must actively engage your abdominals, simply going through the motion without engaging your abdominal wall means you're missing the mark.**

My Conclusion: **Visible ABS requires a combination of disciplined eating, practical training, and low body fat. There's no magic formula, just consistent effort and a focus on sustainable practices. You can achieve a strong, defined *center* core (ABS) with patience and the right strategy.**

Abdominal Obesity

It poses several health risks:

1. Heart Disease: Increases risk due to inflammation, high blood pressure, and cholesterol.

2. Type 2 Diabetes: Causes insulin resistance, raising blood sugar.

3. High Blood Pressure: Affects the body's ability to regulate blood pressure.

4. Fatty Liver Disease: Leads to liver inflammation and potential failure.

5. Sleep Apnea: Increases the likelihood of interrupted breathing during sleep.

6. Cancer: Linked to higher risks of certain cancers like colorectal and breast cancer.

7. Promotes chronic inflammation, worsening various health conditions.

8. Reduced Life Expectancy: Increases risk of premature death due to heart disease and diabetes.

9. Metabolic Syndrome: A cluster of conditions that elevate the risk of heart disease and stroke.

10. Joint Problems: Excess fat strains joints, leading to conditions like osteoarthritis.

Prevention involves a healthy diet, regular exercise, stress management, and avoiding excessive alcohol and smoking.

The Truth About Belly Fat Loss

Getting rid of stubborn belly fat isn't about endless crunches—it's largely about Calories in versus calories out. **You can't spot-reduce fat** in any part of your body. Losing belly fat requires an overall fat-burning approach that targets your entire body.

When it comes to burning belly fat, abdominal exercises alone won't get the job done because they burn very few calories. Instead, **focus on compound movements like squats, push-ups, rows, and steady-state cardio,** which are more effective for fat loss. **However, this doesn't mean ab exercises don't have value. They are essential for improving core strength and mobility, but won't directly melt belly fat.**

Final tips for Abdominal Exercises:

1. Consistency: Ab exercises are essential for building core strength and supporting internal organs. Aim to work your ABS a few times a week, or even daily if your fitness level allows. It's important not to neglect this part of your workout.

2. Hack for Helping to firm Your Abs: You can add a simple method to *help* firm over time. I had my sister do this decades ago: at every red light (safely, of course): contract your muscles for 5–10 seconds as if you're bracing for a light punch. Don't suck in your stomach; **firmly engage/contract your ABS** and don't forget to breathe. This won't give you a six-pack, but it can help firm it; 3 months for her.

3. Add Resistance: To develop more visible ABS, you must incorporate resistance into your abdominal exercises. This helps thicken and shape your muscles, giving you a more defined look.

4. Engage Your ABS During Daily Activities: You can also engage your ABS during everyday movements. For instance, when doing bicep curls, squats, or overhead presses, tighten your stomach as if bracing for a punch. This will help support

your core, protect your lower back, prevent hyperextension, and improve overall posture and body stability.

In summary, while abdominal exercises are valuable for strengthening your core, **fat loss primarily stems from compound resistance movements, cardiovascular exercise and walking [read WALKING SECTION in this book]**. Remain consistent with your abdominal exercises and gradually incorporate resistance for more noticeable results.

Exercising accounts for only 20% of your weight-loss strategy, while nutrition makes up 80%.

> "The Greater Your Muscle Density, The More Calories Your Body Burns—Even At REST."

Steady-state cardio: like walking, can help with belly fat, but it is more effective when combined with strength training and proper nutrition.

Visceral Fat

What Is Visceral Fat? Visceral fat is body fat stored deep within the abdominal cavity, surrounding vital organs like the liver, pancreas, and intestines. Unlike subcutaneous fat (which sits under the skin), you can't pinch visceral fat, but it's the most dangerous type.

Why Is Visceral Fat Dangerous?

Excess visceral fat is strongly linked to:

- Heart disease

- Type 2 diabetes

- Stroke

- High blood pressure

- Insulin resistance

- Certain cancers

- Fatty liver disease

It increases **inflammatory hormones** and interferes with **normal hormone function**, accelerating aging and chronic disease risk.

How to Reduce Visceral Fat (Science-Backed Strategies)

1. Prioritize Protein & Fiber
- High-protein diets help preserve muscle and burn more fat, including visceral fat.

- Soluble fiber (found in oats, avocados, beans, flaxseeds) reduces belly fat by slowing digestion and regulating blood sugar.

2. Limit Added Sugars & Refined Carbs
- Fructose and refined carbs spike insulin and encourage fat storage—especially in the abdominal area.

- Cut out sugary drinks, pastries, white bread, and excess processed foods.

3. Engage in Strength & HIIT Workouts
- Resistance training builds muscle, which boosts metabolism and helps reduce visceral fat.

- High-Intensity Interval Training (HIIT) is especially effective for burning deep belly fat.

4. Sleep & Stress Management
- **Poor sleep and high stress** increase cortisol, a hormone that drives visceral fat gain.

- Aim for **7–9 hours of quality sleep** and use stress-reducing practices like deep breathing, walking, or meditation.

5. Intermittent Fasting (IF) Can Help

- IF may improve insulin sensitivity and reduce visceral fat by enhancing fat metabolism.

- Common approach: **16:8 fasting window** (16 hours fasting, 8 hours eating).

How to Know If You Have Too Much Visceral Fat

- Waist measurement is a simple indicator:

    - Women: >35 inches (88 cm)

    - Men: >40 inches (102 cm)

- **CT scans or DEXA scans** offer precise measurement but are rarely necessary for general health improvement.

In Summary

- Visceral fat is silent but dangerous.

- You can't spot-reduce it—but a combination of diet, resistance training, and lifestyle change can reduce it significantly.

- The goal is not just looking leaner—it's living longer and healthier.

More Sweat, Burn More Fat?

Sweating doesn't directly indicate fat loss; it's a natural cooling mechanism, and the amount varies by person. Some people sweat intensely, even slowly, while others barely sweat during heavy workouts.

My Experience

During my bodybuilding days, I achieved roughly 7-8% body fat without doing any cardio. My fat loss came entirely from intense weightlifting:

- 12–16 sets per body part, twice a week.

- 2+ hours per session with high intensity.

- This slightly demonstrates that you can lose fat without sweat or do cardio if your workouts are regular and demanding. *That said, I believe I would have appeared leaner and more vascular if I had incorporated cardio*; nevertheless, pushing your body through resistance training burns many calories, not so much during the actual training but in the days following.

Weight Training:

- Intense weightlifting and HIIT exercises create a significant calorie burn during and after exercise through **EPOC** (Excess Post-Exercise Oxygen Consumption). This effect can last for 24– 48 hours or produce a 6% to 15% increase in overall calories.

- The key is pushing your muscles to their limit safely, which requires energy for recovery.

Cardio:

- To improve cardio endurance, aim for at least 20 minutes of consistent activity.

- **Interval training** (especially high-intensity interval training, HIIT) can be *more time-efficient* for fat loss than steady cardio. Studies show it burns significant calories in less time and produces greater **EPOC** (excess post-exercise oxygen consumption), which modestly elevates metabolic rate for hours after.

- **However**, total fat loss still depends on overall calorie balance (diet + exercise). Intervals are not automatically "more effective" for everyone — they're more efficient, but steady continuous training can be equally effective when done longer.

Sweating and Calorie Burn
- Sweating doesn't necessarily mean you're burning more calories or losing more fat. Factors such as workout intensity, effort, and individual physiology play a bigger role.

- You can burn fat and improve fitness even with minimal sweating if the workout is effective.

Bottom Line:
- Fat loss comes from consistent, intense efforts, whether through weightlifting, interval training, or a combination of both.

- Sweating is simply a byproduct for some; it's not a measure of workout success.

- **Focus on progressive overload** and sticking to your routine rather than sweating as an indicator of effectiveness.

Disclaimer: I'm not a doctor; this is based on over 50 years of training experience. Always consult a healthcare professional to understand your specific condition and limitations.

Chapter 11
STRONG MOTHERS

> She is clothed with strength and dignity, and she laughs without fear of the future. She speaks with wisdom, and faithful instruction is on her tongue. She watches over the affairs of her household and does not eat the bread of idleness. Her children arise and call her blessed; her husband also, and he praises her: "Many women do noble things, but you surpass them all." Charm is deceptive, and beauty is fleeting, but a woman who fears the Lord is to be praised. Honor her for all that her hands have done, and let her works bring her praise at the city gate. -*Proverbs 31:25–31 NIV*

Too often, mothers may feel guilty for taking time to go to the gym, as if it's selfish. **That couldn't be further from the truth!**

The stronger and healthier a mother is, the better she can care for her family, including aging relatives and growing children. **Self-care isn't selfish; it's essential.**

The challenge is often time. Many women, especially mothers, struggle to carve out even a small part of the day for themselves, and when they do, they may feel guilty. However, prioritizing your health sets the foundation for everything else. The key is to find a workout you enjoy; it doesn't have to be a grueling boot camp that leaves you drained. Furthermore, extreme, unsustainable diets only set you up to fail.

There's a balance: choose an exercise routine you enjoy, one that includes resistance training, and pair it with realistic nutrition habits. Resistance training has been proven time and again to aid in managing stress, anxiety, emotional health, and overall resilience.

> **Nutrition is equally important.** Countless studies show that mothers often influence the eating and fitness habits of the entire household. When mom is active and eats well, the rest of the family tends to follow.

So, find a workout you look forward to. Include strength training as your foundation and add some cardio you enjoy—whether it's speed walking, biking, or dancing. If you're unsure where to start, seek a knowledgeable trainer who understands women's unique needs.

With resistance training, women can double their strength in a year. Most gains occur in the first 3–6 months due to improved nerve-muscle coordination. Consistency and progressive overload are essential.

> **You deserve to feel strong, capable, and healthy for your family and yourself.**

Will Women Get Bulky?

Most women can lift weights without worrying about looking masculine. Developing a bulky physique typically requires specific genetics, very intense training, and in *some* cases, steroid use. For most, **strength training builds lean muscle, improves tone, and boosts overall fitness without bulk.**

Muscle development varies greatly by body type. Just like in professional bodybuilding, Frank Zane and Arnold Schwarzenegger had completely different physiques. Zane was known for his aesthetic, lean, symmetrical build, while Arnold had a larger, more muscular frame with a powerful chest. Despite both being elite athletes, their genetics and structure shaped how their bodies responded to training. Arnold couldn't achieve Zane's slim, tapered look, and Zane couldn't develop the mass and bulk of Arnold, no matter how they trained.

In the same way, each person's training results are influenced by their unique body type, not just their workout routine. **Practical training isn't about endless hours in the gym; it's about being present, intentional, and fully engaged.**

- Own your space and master the **mind-muscle connection** to unlock real progress. **Lift pure**—it's not just about moving weight, but activating muscle fibers. *Stimulate,* **don't annihilate. Form and precision always come first.** Clear out negativity before every set, give it your all, and promise yourself you'll push beyond your limits to become your best.

- When you train, own the moment. Focus. Don't drift. Work it, kill it, change your life.

The idea that most women will become "bulky" from lifting weights is a common misconception. Here's a logical breakdown of the factors involved:

> **Factors Influencing Muscle Growth:** Research shows that women need to engage in intense resistance training to build significant muscle mass. This training includes heavy loads (typically 65–85% of their one-repetition max), high training volume (multiple sets per muscle group per week), and sufficient intensity to reach near-muscular fatigue.

Supporting science-based details:

Training volume (sets × reps × weight) is a major driver of hypertrophy (Schoenfeld, 2010).

- **Heavy resistance** (65–85% of 1RM) effectively recruits muscle fibers needed for growth.

- **Training intensity** close to failure is important to maximize muscle fiber recruitment (Schoenfeld et al., 2016).

- Women generally **recover faster** and may handle slightly more volume per session compared to men (Simao et al., 2012).

Genetics: Genetics plays a significant role in muscle development. Some individuals naturally have more muscle mass or develop it faster due to their DNA. Example: You could have siblings with the same coach, and training regimen, yet one may have a more muscular physique while the other is leaner, highlighting the influence of genetics.

Reference-Backed Claims:

- **Schoenfeld, B. J. (2010, 2016):** Volume and intensity are primary drivers of hypertrophy.

- **Simao et al. (2012):** Women can often tolerate higher training volume and recover faster than men.

- **Boutcher, S. H. (2011):** HIIT improves fat loss and lean mass retention.

- **American Council on Exercise (ACE):** Discusses muscle tone, fat loss, and strength training benefits.

- **Phillips et al.:** Protein utilization and anabolic resistance with aging.

- **Leucine research (Tipton & Wolfe):** Leucine threshold needed to trigger muscle protein synthesis

Steroids & Enhancements:
- Many professional bodybuilders (male and female) use steroids, which significantly enhance muscle growth.

- Women who appear extremely muscular, resembling men in size, may *possibly* use anabolic steroids or other performance-enhancing drugs. In contrast, women in fitness competitions, such as those in bikini or fitness categories, generally avoid such substances, instead focusing on achieving a natural muscle tone.

Three Powerful Training Methods—Different Tools for Different Goals

1. Circuit Training
This method involves rotating through a series of exercises—*typically* 5 to 10—with minimal rest between stations. It's time-efficient and keeps your heart rate elevated, making it great for fat loss, muscular endurance, and general conditioning. Loads are usually moderate, and the focus is on movement rather than maximum intensity or muscle overload.

My personal format for active older adults: 4–5 exercises, 3–4 rounds, alternating *push/pull/lower/core pattern*s; that is now supported by both clinical practice and current older-adult training guidelines.

2. HIIT (High-Intensity Interval Training)
HIIT alternates short bursts of intense effort (like sprints or fast-paced bodyweight exercises) with periods of rest or low-intensity movement. It's designed to improve cardiovascular health, burn fat, and enhance athletic performance. Work periods are explosive and fast-paced, pushing your heart rate to near max levels. HIIT is not the same as resistance

training and won't build much muscle, but it's effective for metabolic conditioning and fat loss.

3. Resistance Training

This includes lifting weights or using resistance bands with structured sets, reps, and rest. It's the most effective method for building muscle, increasing strength, and improving overall body composition. Many women worry this will lead to a bulky look, but in reality, it builds lean, toned muscle and supports long-term fat loss. For those who *do* want to build more visible muscle—awesome. That's a powerful and valid goal.

Science-Backed Points

- Muscle tone results from increased muscle definition coupled with lower body fat levels (American Council on Exercise).

- Building significant muscle mass typically requires high training volume, progressive overload, an *appropriate* caloric *surplus*, and long-term consistency.

- Most women lack the testosterone levels required for easy or rapid muscle growth (Schoenfeld, 2010).

- HIIT and circuit training effectively preserve lean mass while promoting fat loss (Boutcher, 2011).

Muscle Tone Vs. Bulk

- Women respond to training differently based on individual genetics and body composition—some may build visible muscle tone more easily, while others stay lean despite similar routines. This is also true for men.

- Lower testosterone levels in women naturally limit the potential for excessive muscle growth.

- Body type—whether ectomorph, mesomorph, or endomorph—plays a significant role in how a person develops muscle and stores fat.

Why Women Should Lift Weights:

Strength & Health Benefits:
Weightlifting helps build stronger bones, improves metabolism, and enhances overall strength. It shapes and tones muscles, creating a leaner and more athletic physique.

No Need to Fear Bulk:
Unless you lift extremely heavy weights for many sets with high volume and train like bodybuilders, women will typically not become "bulky."

Female Testosterone

1. **Yes** — Women naturally generate testosterone, but typically in much lesser quantities than men. Even at these reduced levels, testosterone is crucial for women's fitness, energy, and general health.

2. **Why** Testosterone Matters for Exercise

- Testosterone promotes lean muscle growth and aids the body's recovery process after workouts.

- It affects how and where the body stores fat, influencing physical appearance and weight management.

- Healthy testosterone levels also contribute to improved energy, focus, and motivation during workouts, while low levels can make exercise feel more difficult.

- Additionally, testosterone helps maintain bone density, which becomes increasingly important as we age.

What Affects Testosterone in Women
- Testosterone levels naturally decline over time, particularly after menopause.

- Some forms of birth control can reduce testosterone production.

- High stress levels, due to elevated cortisol, can also suppress it.
- Overtraining or inadequate nutrition can disrupt hormonal balance.
- Certain medical conditions like PCOS may lead to higher testosterone levels.

4. Can Women Naturally Boost Their Testosterone Levels?
- Yes. Strength training with heavier weights or almost any resistance exercises help stimulate testosterone production, *not necessarily bulk*.
- Getting quality sleep, managing stress, and eating a diet rich in healthy fats, such as avocados, nuts, and olive oil, all support hormone health.
- Nutrients like zinc and vitamin D also play a role in maintaining balanced testosterone levels.

Perimenopause & Menopause (40 & Beyond)

Women entering perimenopause and menopause experience hormonal and physiological changes that impact overall health and body composition. A proactive fitness and wellness strategy can significantly ease the transition and support long-term vitality.

Physiological Changes and Health Risks

1. **Bone Health** – Bone density declines rapidly during this transition, increasing the risk of osteoporosis and fractures. Strength training is crucial for maintaining strong bones.

2. **Muscle Mass and Fat Gain** – Without regular resistance training, muscle mass decreases while fat accumulation becomes easier, leading to metabolic changes.

3. **Increased Health Risks** – This period is associated with a higher risk of diabetes and heart disease, making physical activity essential for long-term health.

4. **Common Symptoms** – Hot flashes are one of the most well-known symptoms; regular exercise can help manage them.

Exercise Recommendations

1. **Strength Training** – Resistance training is essential for bone density, muscle retention, and metabolic health.

2. **Functional Fitness**—Incorporate flexibility exercises, yoga, Pilates, exercises that simulate everyday movements, dynamic stretching, and foam rolling to improve body awareness, muscle synergy, and joint alignment.

3. **Balance Training** – This is important for fall prevention, especially as we age. Balance declines over time, but targeted exercises can help maintain stability.

4. **Cardio & Recovery** – Include cardiovascular exercise while allowing rest days between strength sessions for optimal recovery.

Exercise caution and avoid high-impact or technical movements (e.g., Olympic lifts) unless you are adequately trained. Proper form and a structured program are essential for injury prevention.

Final Thoughts: Strength training and balance exercises are essential for long-term health. Swimming and machine-based resistance training are good alternatives. If needed, seek guidance from a qualified trainer.

Menopause & Protein

What the Science Really Says

1. **The 30g Protein Myth:** "The 30 g-protein-per-meal guideline comes from MPS research in younger adults, where muscle synthesis plateaus around 20–30 g of high-quality protein. Because menopause can bring hormonal changes and reduced muscle responsiveness, some experts propose slightly higher doses (e.g. up to 30–40 g) per meal—but evidence is preliminary.

2. **The Truth About the "Anabolic Window"**

    - The idea of a **strict 45-minute window** post-workout is outdated.

    - Research shows the muscle-building window actually lasts **2–3 hours**.

- What matters most is your **total daily protein intake**, not just what you eat right after a workout.

- That said, eating protein **within a couple of hours** post-workout is still a **smart habit**.

3. Protein Needs During Menopause:

Lower estrogen levels may impair muscle maintenance and reduce protein utilization. To counteract that, many experts suggest post-menopausal women aim for **1.0 to 1.5 g of protein per kilogram of body weight per day**, especially when doing resistance training. Distribute that across **3 to 4 meals**, targeting **25 to 35 g of high-quality protein per meal** with emphasis on **2.5 to 3 g leucine** per meal. Focus on *leucine-rich sources such as eggs, dairy, poultry, fish, lean meats, or plant-based blends that are fortified with leucine.*

> **Total protein intake and consistency throughout the day are far more important than exact timing.**

Chapter 12
SENIOR EXERCISES

Getting Started Safely

Medical Clearance: Before beginning any fitness program, always consult your physician, especially if you have:
- Heart conditions
- Previous injuries
- Past surgeries
- Ongoing medical concerns

Assess Your Current Ability
Ask yourself:
- Can I get up from the floor quickly without using my hands?
- Can I walk around the block at a steady pace while maintaining a conversation?
- How do I feel during daily tasks like climbing stairs, getting out of a car, or pushing a shopping cart?

Exercise Recommendations: Aerobic Activity: Aim for at least 150 minutes per week of moderate-intensity aerobic exercise (e.g., walking, biking, water aerobics), with your doctor's approval.

Strength Training for Active Older Adults

- Train each major muscle group 2–3 nonconsecutive days per week.

- Use a weight that allows 8–15 reps per set with good form, with 10–12 as a strong default.

- If heavier loading isn't possible, lighter weights with 15–20 reps work for maintenance or endurance.

- Avoid loads that force broken form or joint pain; under supervision, loads ≥75% 1RM may be used safely in many older adults.

- Practical structure: 4–5 exercises per session, 3–4 rounds (sets), rotating push/pull/lower/core patterns.

- Progress gradually by increasing load or reps as tolerated, adjusting for recovery, pain, and outcomes.

- Seek out a knowledgeable coach or trainer with years of experience working with adults over 50.

Other Exercises and Tools
Bodyweight Exercises
Low-impact and joint-friendly, requiring minimal equipment:
- Modified push-ups (wall, countertop *safely*, back of a couch, or on knees)
- Chair squats or bodyweight squats
- Lunges with support if needed
- Planks, modify as needed
- Step-ups on aerobic step, or side steps for mobility

Resistance Bands
- Provide controlled resistance
- Improve strength and balance
- Ideal for joint limitations

Machines and Dumbbells
- Machines with adjustable or guided motion (e.g., cable machines) offer safer control
- Dumbbells are effective but require good form
- **Avoid machines that force unnatural joint angles**

Leg Strength Focus

- Leg press machines with **proper back support** are safer than barbell squats (which I emphatically do *not* recommend).
- Hack squat machines **with full back support** reduce spine pressure, not with the padded arms.
- Dumbbell squats, held hanging or at shoulder height, are great for balance and strength.
- Modified Deadlifts
  - Use light weights and limited range of motion
  - Stop at mid-shin height
  - Elevate weights on aerobic steps to avoid excess bending

Progressing Safely

Start with movements you can perform comfortably and with good form. Examples include:
- Sit-to-stand chair exercises
- Standing marches
- Resistance band arm raises
- Modified jumping jacks (stepping side to side)

Gradually increase the challenge as you progress:
- Add repetitions or sets
- Introduce light resistance
- Safely increase range of motion

Exercise Classes & Sports for Those New to Fitness

Emphasizing safety, gradual progress, and enjoyment; perfect starting points for building confidence and mobility

Gentle Group Classes (Low Impact)
- Chair Yoga – Boosts flexibility and relaxation without strain
- SilverSneakers® – Specially designed for older adults; often free with insurance
- Beginner Tai Chi – Improves balance, coordination, and mental clarity
- Water Aerobics – Joint-friendly cardio and strength training in the pool
- Stretch & Balance Classes – Reduces fall risk and increases mobility

Strength and Functional Training; Helps improve daily function, independence, and metabolism:
- Resistance Band Training – Easy on joints but highly effective
- Light Dumbbell Circuits – Focus on form, control, and posture
- Functional Fitness Classes – Mimic real-life movements (sit-to-stand, reaching, stepping)
- TRX for Seniors – Assisted bodyweight moves to improve strength and balance

Cardio-Friendly & Social Activities; Encourages heart health and community involvement:
- Walking Clubs – Safe, scalable, and social
- Pickleball (Beginner Clinics) – Low-impact and fun, growing rapidly among seniors
- Low-Impact Zumba (Zumba Gold) – Dance-style cardio adapted for older adults

- Cycling (Recumbent or Stationary Bikes) – Great for knees and endurance

Mind-Body Integration: Builds internal strength, body awareness, and calm:
- Beginner Pilates (Mat or Reformer) – Core strength and flexibility
- Qigong – A more meditative movement art, very beginner-friendly
- Breathing & Meditation Classes – Especially for stress relief and cognitive health

Other Fun & Functional Sports:
- Bowling (with lighter balls) – Social and coordination-based
- Golf (or Mini Golf) – Walking, swinging, and strategy
- Dancing (Ballroom, Line Dancing) – Great for brain, heart, and social life

What to Avoid:
- High-impact, fast-paced movements like burpees or box jumps
- Trainers who push aggressive or unsafe workouts
- Ignoring pain or pushing through discomfort

Embracing the Power of Movement: With the right approach, the human body shows remarkable resilience—even in the 80s and 90s. The outdated belief that aging means slowing down or becoming sedentary is being replaced by powerful examples of active older adults.

It's never too late to start. Even those who've remained inactive for years can experience incredible improvements. At our studio, we've seen people in their 50s, 60s, and 70s—many new to structured exercise—make life-changing progress in just six to nine months. Energy improves. Mobility returns. Confidence grows.

Prioritizing Safety and Individual Needs

Every body is unique. Fitness routines should be tailored to individual history, injuries, and experience level.
- A 60-year-old former athlete will differ from someone starting fresh.
- Past injuries (like knee replacements or sciatica) require adjustments to prevent aggra-

vation.

• Medical devices like pacemakers may also affect workout choices—consult your doctor.

Form Over Ego: Proper technique is essential. As we age, controlled movement protects joints and enhances gains. It's not about lifting heavy—it's about moving well. Even modified movements—like partial squats, gentle leg presses, or shortened-range deadlifts—can build meaningful strength.

Beyond the Weights

Success in fitness depends on more than just exercise. Key influences include:

• Diet: Nutrition fuels muscle growth and recovery
• Rest: Sleep and rest are critical for repair
• Stress: Chronic stress affects hormones and slows progress

Training Smart-Mobility Over Muscle Mass

Intensity with Intention: Older adults should avoid pushing to complete muscle failure, unlike younger or highly trained athletes. Instead, they should aim to stop 2–3 reps before that point. This approach helps maintain control, reduce fatigue, and lower the risk of injury.

Increasing workout intensity can be beneficial, but it should always serve a purpose, such as preparing for a charity walk or achieving a personal milestone. Any increase should be made gradually and with professional guidance.

For older adults, transitioning from bodybuilding-style training to functional movement offers lasting benefits. Consider Bruce Lee—his emphasis on flexibility, balance, and real-world movement not only made him strong but also fluid and efficient. He utilized machines and isometrics but always prioritized functional strength.

In contrast, heavy lifting that focuses purely on muscle size often adds unnecessary stress and may not translate well to everyday functions. **Building a body that moves well and feels good is far more valuable.**

More Than Muscle: The True Benefits of Exercise

Improved Mobility and Balance: Regular exercise enhances flexibility, coordination, and balance, reducing the risk of falls and maintaining independence in daily life.

Increased Strength and Energy Levels: Building muscle density and improving cardiovascular fitness can help combat age-related muscle loss, thereby increasing energy levels and making daily activities more enjoyable and less taxing.

Enhanced Quality of Life: Regular physical activity has been shown to improve mood, reduce stress, and enhance overall well-being, contributing to a higher quality of life and a greater sense of purpose.

A Journey of Lifelong Learning and Adaptation. Embarking on a fitness journey later in life requires a mindful and personalized approach. Working with a qualified fitness trainer experienced in senior fitness can provide valuable guidance, ensuring that your exercise program is safe, effective, and enjoyable.

Prioritize safety and long-term consistency over the pursuit of extreme intensity. Listen to your body, adjust your routine as needed, and celebrate your progress, no matter how small.

Remember, you are never too old to exercise and improve your health. Adopting a proactive and informed approach to fitness can unlock your full potential and allow you to enjoy a vibrant, fulfilling life at almost any age.

Final Thoughts: Elevating Every Rep

The measure of a successful workout isn't how many reps you complete—**it's the quality of each one.**

If your goal is twelve, make each rep count. Focus, breathe, engage. Treat each movement as a reflection of your intent and commitment.

> **Never underestimate the power of mindful execution. When you train with purpose, every rep becomes more than just movement—it becomes a message to your body that you're still in the game.**

Longevity —Thriving: Quality of Life

Longevity isn't just about adding years to life—it's about adding life to those years. Across the globe, particularly in the world's longest-living cultures, people thrive not from high-tech health fads, but from **simple, powerful, natural habits** woven into everyday living. Their strength, balance, endurance, and nourishment support a vibrant, independent life well into old age.

1. Movement Is Medicine

In long-living regions—known as Blue Zones—people don't schedule workouts; they move naturally throughout the day, walk to visit neighbors, garden, carry tools, and climb hills. Movement is part of life—not an event.

This daily motion supports metabolic health, mobility, and muscular function in ways most sedentary lives no longer do.

Walking speed matters. A 2011 JAMA study showed that older adults with slower gait speed had higher mortality, while those who walked faster tended to live longer.[1]

2. Deep Squatting and Longevity

In many rural and tribal cultures—from Asia to South America—people spend hours in a deep squat. It's how they rest, cook, eat, and socialize.

This position keeps the hips, knees, and ankles mobile, the spine aligned, and the lower body strong.

Research supports this. In a study of 2,000 adults aged 51–80, those who could sit and rise from the floor without assistance had significantly lower death rates.[2]

"Deep squatting isn't just primitive—it's preserving." —Kelly Starrett

3. Strength Predicts Survival

Strength isn't just about fitness—it's about freedom. Being able to push, grip, or rise from the floor is linked directly to how long—and how well—you live.

- **Push-ups**: Men who could complete 40 or more had a 96% lower risk of heart events than those who could do fewer than 10.[3]

- **Grip strength**: In a study of 17 countries, weaker grip predicted early death better than high blood pressure.[4]

- **Leg strength**: Essential for preventing falls and maintaining independence. Squats, lunges, and standing movements keep this power intact.

Your strength is your safeguard.

4. VO$_2$ Max: The Oxygen Advantage

VO$_2$ max—your body's ability to use oxygen—is one of the strongest predictors of life expectancy.[5]

Improving it through walking, intervals, or aerobic training doesn't just build stamina—it protects your heart and brain. Even modest gains reduce the risk of early death.

It's never too late to build your oxygen engine.

5. Eat Close to the Source

Those thriving into their 80s and 90s eat real food—whole, unprocessed, and close to how nature made it.

Their diets center on vegetables, fruits, legumes, lean proteins, olive oil, and fermented foods. Meals are simple, intentional, and often shared. In Okinawa, they follow *Hara Hachi Bu*—eating until 80% full.

It's not restriction—it's rhythm.

6. Purpose, Connection, and Joy

Every longevity hotspot shares this: a strong sense of purpose, tight social ties, and spiritual grounding.

Whether it's *ikigai* in Japan or *plan de vida* in Costa Rica, meaning and connection protect against isolation, depression, and decline.

They don't just live long. They live like it matters.

> *The Takeaway: Real health is functional— we train to live fully and freely. Health isn't just about abs or a number on a scale; it's about squatting with ease, walking daily, carrying your groceries, getting off the floor, and holding your grandchild.*

Selected References

1. Studenski, S., et al. (2011). *Gait speed and survival in older adults*. JAMA.

2. Brito, L. B., et al. (2012). *Ability to sit and rise from the floor as a predictor of all-cause mortality*. European Journal of Preventive Cardiology.

3. Yang, J., et al. (2019). *Association Between Push-up Exercise Capacity and Future*

Cardiovascular Events. JAMA Network Open.

4. Leong, D. P., et al. (2015). *Prognostic value of grip strength: PURE study.* The Lancet.

5. Kodama, S., et al. (2009). *Cardiorespiratory fitness as a quantitative predictor of all-cause mortality.* JAMA.

Chapter 13
BEHAVIORAL STRATEGIES

The Psychology Behind Sustainable Change

Set Realistic Goals
Set achievable weight loss targets and track progress.

Plan Meals
Prepare meals in advance to avoid unhealthy choices.

Keep a Food Diary
Track intake, emotions, and hunger to identify patterns.

Find Support
Join a group or find a friend for motivation.

Celebrate Non-Scale Victories
Focus on energy, fitness, and clothing fit—not just the number on the scale.

By understanding triggers, you can stay on track and make lasting, healthy changes.

Triggers To Watch Out For

It's crucial to be aware of the different factors that can affect your weight loss journey. Here are some important points to consider:

Emotional Eating

Trigger: Stress, boredom, sadness, or anxiety.

Strategy: Identify emotional triggers and find alternative coping mechanisms like *proper* guidance in your exercise, meditation, or hobbies.

Environmental Cues

Trigger: Seeing or smelling food, social events, or eating out.

Strategy: Keep healthy snacks available, plan meals in advance, and choose restaurants with healthy options.

Hunger and Cravings

Trigger: Skipping meals, *restrictive* unhealthy dieting, or high-sugar foods.

Strategy: Eat balanced meals with protein, fiber, and healthy fats to stay full longer and avoid extreme hunger.

Social Pressure

Trigger: Friends or family encouraging you to eat more or indulge.

Strategy: Communicate your goals to your social circle and seek support from those who understand your objectives.

Physical Stress & Muscle Adaptation

In weightlifting, resistance causes microscopic tears in muscle fibers. This triggers a repair process where satellite cells fuse to the damaged fibers, increasing muscle size and strength. This process—called hypertrophy—is driven by mechanical tension, metabolic stress, and muscle damage.

The body responds by increasing protein synthesis and releasing growth factors like IGF-1 and testosterone. If the stress becomes excessive (e.g., overtraining), it can lead to chronic inflammation, fatigue, and poor recovery.

Metabolic Stress & Nutritional Adaptation

The body also adapts to dietary stressors like caloric restriction or fasting. Intermittent fasting triggers autophagy—cellular cleanup and renewal—supporting longevity and metabolic health.

Caloric restriction enhances insulin sensitivity and activates pathways like AMPK, which supports fat burning and mitochondrial efficiency. Carbohydrate cycling helps train the body to efficiently use both carbs and fats for fuel.

Psychological Stress & Adaptation

Short-term stress can improve focus, alertness, and energy. When managed well, it strengthens the HPA (hypothalamic-pituitary-adrenal) axis and builds psychological resilience.

But *chronic stress* tells a different story. It elevates cortisol, disrupts sleep, impairs recovery, and promotes muscle breakdown (catabolism).

The Balance of Stress & Recovery

Stress is useful when paired with recovery. This is hormesis—controlled stress followed by recovery leads to growth.

- Too little stress = no progress
- Too much stress = burnout
- The right stress + recovery = transformation

Rewire Your Brain With Self-Talk & Discipline

Finding Your Higher Purpose

Challenges like time constraints, low motivation, health issues, and financial pressure can feel overwhelming. But with purpose and consistency, these can be overcome.

Common Barriers and How to Handle Them:

- **Lack of Time or Energy**

    Carve out time where you can. Even 10 minutes adds up.

- **Health Conditions**

    Modify, don't quit. Movement is medicine.

- **Perfectionism & Negative Self-Talk**

    Progress beats perfection. Talk to yourself with compassion.

- **Lack of Knowledge**

    Please don't complicate it all. Start simple. Walking, light resistance, consistency—that's enough to begin.

Exercise Fuels Emotional Wellness

1. Acknowledge the Challenge
Tough days happen. Show up anyway.

2. Mind-Body Benefits
- Releases endorphins
- Reduces anxiety and depression
- Boosts clarity, confidence, and emotional stability

3. Getting Started
Begin with what you can do. Walking, stretching, even cleaning counts.

4. Make it Social
Group workouts, gym buddies, and fitness classes can boost motivation.

5. Build Your Routine
30 minutes, 3, maybe 4 days a week, is enough to create real change.

6. Face Setbacks with Grace
Off days are part of the journey. Don't let them derail your progress.

7. Don't Wait for Motivation
Discipline backed by purpose will carry you farther.

Staying on Track

1. Know Your Schedule
Workout at the time of day that fits your life. There is no one-size-fits-all.

2. Make It a Priority
Your health is the foundation for everything else. Treat it like a non-negotiable.

3. Kill the Excuses

Short on time? Do what you can: bodyweight workouts, stair climbs, lunchtime walks.

4. Create a Real Routine

Wake up earlier, go straight to the gym after work, or find micro-moments throughout the day to move.

5. Balance with Family Life

Include your family. Walks, hikes, sports—they all count.

6. Maximize Every Opportunity

Use home workouts, work breaks, or standing desks to stay active.

7. Remember: Small Actions Add Up

Little choices become big results over time.

A Higher Purpose Checklist

When motivation fades, purpose keeps you going. Write your "why" and post it where you'll see it daily.

Your reason might be:

- Keeping up with your kids or grandkids

- Feeling more energy and confidence

- Climbing stairs without fatigue

- Improving blood pressure or reversing diabetes

- Honoring your body as a temple of strength and resilience

Second-Person Self-Talk

Speaking to yourself as "you" instead of "I" boosts focus, discipline, and resilience. It's like having a coach in your head.

Use It Like This:

Before a challenge: "You've done the work. You're ready."

Under pressure: "You've been here before. Breathe. You've got this."
When building habits: "You follow through even when it's hard."
At night: "You made progress today. You'll build on it tomorrow."

Final Thoughts: You don't need perfection. You need movement, purpose, and consistency. Small steps lead to massive change when taken with intention. Show up, stay grounded, and believe in your ability to grow—physically, mentally, emotionally.

Chapter 14
NUTRITION — Eat Like Your Life Depends on it

Welcome to a new beginning—a new way of thinking about your health, your body, and your future. This section isn't about rigid rules or trendy fads. It's grounded in timeless nutritional principles, not prescriptions. You won't find strict meal plans here. Instead, you'll discover practical, flexible strategies designed to help you make confident, lasting choices. Nutrition isn't just about what you eat—it's about building a respectful, sustainable relationship with food; one that fuels your goals and honors the body you're working hard to strengthen.

Your path is your own. What follows are time-tested approaches centered around real, whole foods: **lean proteins to help build strength, vegetables to nourish your cells, healthy fats to sharpen your mind, and smart carbs to fuel your day.** This isn't a diet manual—it's a launchpad, drawn from over fifty years of experience in fitness and wellness. Clear. Adaptable. Empowering. Because real change doesn't come all at once—it happens one meal, one choice, one step at a time. You weren't made to be average. You were made for more. **Fuel your body. Fuel your mind. Fuel your purpose.**

The Fuel Behind Your Transformation

When it comes to nutrition, there's no one-size-fits-all solution. Some plans are overly simplistic; others feel unnecessarily complex. The truth lies somewhere in the middle—and it begins with starting *somewhere*. You don't need to commit to one approach forever. What you begin with may evolve into something better suited for the long haul.

Maybe you kick things off with a low-carb plan like keto or Atkins, to establish your eating patterns and reduce cravings. But over time, something more balanced—like a Mediterranean-style approach or simply focusing on whole, unprocessed foods—might better match your lifestyle. If you *love* carbs, keto might not be the best fit. If you prefer a less restrictive way of eating with room for variety, that shift can make all the difference. Whether it's intermittent fasting, South Beach, Atkins, or something else—**they've all worked for someone. What matters most is what works *for you*.**

> The key is to choose a direction you can realistically maintain. The best diet in the world won't work if it doesn't fit your life. This isn't just about short-term weight loss—it's about building a way of eating that supports your body, your energy, and your goals over time.

Let me be upfront—this isn't a recipe book. You won't find daily meal plans or detailed breakdowns for breakfast, lunch, and dinner. That's not the purpose of this section. There are plenty of excellent books that focus solely on that—and I encourage you to explore them if that's what you need.

What I'm offering here is something *different*, and in many ways more important: direction. You'll find clear, easy-to-follow outlines of proven dietary approaches—not to overwhelm or restrict you, but to help you discover what works best for your body, your lifestyle, and your goals.

I'm not here to hand you a rigid formula. I'm here to help you find a path you can actually follow—one that feels sustainable, realistic, and effective for the long term. *"Most people drop off within the first two to three months—often within the first 30 to 60 days—because they chose a plan they couldn't sustain."*

So, have grace with yourself. Choose progress over perfection. Pick a path that challenges you but also fits your lifestyle. This is your journey, and lasting change starts with a plan you can actually live with.

If you walk away from this section with a better understanding of the options, and the confidence to choose the one that feels right for you, then I've done what I came here to do. My hope—my prayer—is that these words offer not just information, but true guidance.

> **Everyone's Needs Are Different—Check With a Qualified Nutritionist or Dietitian**
>
> As a certified nutritionist, I also heavily draw upon five decades of experience in fitness and research. That said, nutrition isn't one-size-fits-all. Use this information as a guide, and be sure to consult a qualified professional who understands your individual needs.

Calories In vs. Out Isn't the Whole Picture

Calories do matter, but consuming 5,000 calories of even protein a day won't work if your goal is a 1,500-calorie diet—there's a fine line between quality and quantity. That's why tracking your intake and focusing on balanced nutrition is key.

> Tracking your **macros—protein, carbs, and fats**—is essential if you want real results. It gives you a clear picture of what you're actually eating, not just guessing. Start by using a simple app on your phone or even a notepad. At first, it may feel like a chore, but after a few months, it becomes second nature. You'll be able to eyeball a plate and know where you stand. Above all, getting enough protein is key. Without tracking consistently—especially early on—it's hard to stay on target. I did it myself during my bodybuilding days, and I can tell you: it makes all the difference.

Aim to **balance proteins, carbohydrates, and fats**. Good protein sources include tofu, chicken (both breasts and thighs), lean cuts of pork and beef, duck, and fish.

> **When Starting Your New Meal Plan, It's Essential To Treat It Like Following A Recipe. If You Don't Measure Your Ingredients Correctly, The Final Dish Won't Turn Out The Way You Intended. The Same Goes For Your Macros.**

Protein should be your top priority. I know it can be tough to hit 20, 30, even 35 grams of protein per meal depending on your plan. I won't argue that—it *is* hard; so weigh everything out and measure everything. Use a tracking app if you so desire. When I started doing this years ago I was just as strict, and could eventually look at a plate and estimate the protein, carbs, sugar, and fat content by sight. Back when I began my fitness journey in the 70s, there were no app trackers. Heck, there weren't even cell phones. But that diligence paid off. I learned by doing, and you will too. Treat your nutrition like a recipe—measure it, learn it, and soon you'll develop an instinct for what's right and what's not.

- Your #1 focus is **protein intake**. Let the other macros (carbs and fat) go up and down *a bit*—it doesn't matter much for many diets, <u>***unless you're on a specific low-carb diet***</u>.

> Back in the '60s and '70s, both low-carb and low-fat diets had their moment—and both worked for some people and failed for others. That's because there is no one-size-fits-all approach. Everyone's body is different. Energy levels vary, and so does metabolism. As I explain throughout this book, you have to find what works for you, and that often means experimenting. If your goal is weight loss, the first priority is usually keeping carbs low—unless you're extremely active, like a long-distance runner or someone training hard in the gym for 90 minutes a day, similar to a semi-professional athlete.

- Choose **real whole foods**. i.e. "Eat to As Close as God Made It, If Man Touched It, They Messed It Up!"

- **Avoid processed food,** which is **73 %** of grocery shelves!

- **Avoiding simple carbs** to prevent insulin spikes is a wise choice for maintaining stable energy levels and overall health. The body quickly breaks down simple carbs, which can cause rapid increases in blood sugar. Stick with complex, low-glycemic carbs.

- You *CAN* **workout on an Empty Stomach to get in the Fat Zone** if you *exercise for less than one hour* – confirm with your coach.

- Cheat *meals*, not days – but not at beginning of your diet.

- Be watchful of Deli Meat, **sodium is off the charts.**

- **Don't "drink" your calories;** and limit fruit juice; **eat the whole fruit instead** plus you will get the fiber.

- **Read Labels**: Look for hidden sugars in ingredient lists. Avoid high amounts of sugar, high fructose corn syrup, or refined flour. Keep any sugar grams in the single digits **under 25-50 gms.** *daily for weight loss or diabetes.*

- **Calorie Cycle:** You can eat a bit more on training days. *Pray or ponder when you sit to eat what you want the food to do in your body and observe what you're eating to help you reach your healthy goals.*

> **Rehydrate Every Morning:** Drink roughly 12–20 oz of water upon waking—for the rest of your life. Your body is about 70% water, so meet your daily needs. Remember: around 20% of water intake comes from food.

- Flushes your kidneys
- Aids digestion
- Supports circulation and lymphatic flow
- Lubricates joints
- Helps organs and cells function properly
- Flushes toxins from the body
- Cleanses the bowels

Protein Estimation, General Rule of Thumb: Most raw animal proteins (red meat, fish, chicken, eggs) average 5–8 grams of protein per ounce, or 4–5 grams per egg. Over the past four decades, I've relied on 5 grams per ounce as a simple, quick estimate. Over time, this balances out across meals and food types.

> **Everyone's Needs Are Different—Check With a Qualified Nutritionist or Dietitian.**

Macronutrients

Every individual is unique. The following is a general outline of daily macronutrient ranges, expressed as total daily calorie intake percentages. These recommendations are geared toward men and women who exercise regularly (about 2–3 hours of resistance training per week) and are either just beginning a fitness journey or rebuilding a fitness base.

These numbers are not used for competitive athletes, bodybuilders, or those with specialized needs.

I strongly recommend consulting a registered dietitian or nutritionist for a personalized approach. The values below are supported by trusted sources, including the Mayo Clinic, and should be adjusted based on your energy levels, body composition goals, and overall health.

Recommended Macronutrient Breakdown

As % of total daily calories:

- **Protein: 15–25%** — Supports muscle repair, metabolism, and appetite control. Higher intake (20–25%) may benefit fat loss or strength goals.

- **Carbohydrates: 45–55%** — Primary energy source for daily function and physical activity. Can be adjusted upward with higher training volumes.

- **Fats: 25–30%** — Essential for hormone production and crucial for cell structure, brain function, and sustained energy.

Daily Fiber Intake – Supports digestion, blood sugar control, and satiety:
- Men: 30–38 grams

- Women: 21–25 grams

Protein-Rich Food Examples:

- **Chicken breast (100 g)** — 31 g protein, 3.6 g fat, 0 g carbs
- **Egg (1 large)** — 6 g protein, 5 g fat, 0.6 g carbs
- **Ground beef (85–92% lean, 100 g)** — 26–28 g protein, 17 g fat, 0 g carbs
- **Pork tenderloin (100 g)** — 26–29 g protein, 3–4 g fat, 0 g carbs
- **Turkey breast (100 g)** — 29 g protein, 1 g fat, 0 g carbs
- **Salmon (100 g)** — 25 g protein, 13 g fat, 0 g carbs
- **Tuna (canned in water, 100 g)** — 23 g protein, 1 g fat, 0 g carbs
- **Carbohydrate-Rich Food Examples**
- **Brown rice (cooked, 1 cup)** — 5 g protein, 1.8 g fat, 45 g carbs
- **Oats (rolled, dry, ½ cup)** — 5 g protein, 3 g fat, 27 g carbs
- **Whole wheat bread (1 slice)** — 4 g protein, 1 g fat, 12 g carbs
- **Sweet potato (1 medium, baked)** — 2 g protein, 0 g fat, 24 g carbs
- **Banana (1 medium)** — 1 g protein, 0 g fat, 27 g carbs
- **Apple (1 medium)** — 0.5 g protein, 0.3 g fat, 25 g carbs

Fat-Rich Whole Foods (Healthy Sources):

- **Avocados**
  Primary Fat: Monounsaturated
  Macronutrient Focus: Healthy fats, fiber

- **Olives / Olive Oil**

Primary Fat: Monounsaturated
Macronutrient Focus: Healthy fats

- **Nuts** *(almonds, walnuts, pistachios, pecans)*
  Primary Fat: Mono- and polyunsaturated
  Macronutrient Focus: Healthy fats, protein

- **Seeds** *(chia, flax, pumpkin, sunflower)*
  Primary Fat: Polyunsaturated
  Macronutrient Focus: Healthy fats, some protein

- **Nut Butters** *(natural, unsweetened)*
  Primary Fat: Monounsaturated
  Macronutrient Focus: Healthy fats, protein

- **Fatty Fish** *(salmon, sardines, mackerel)*
  Primary Fat: Omega-3 polyunsaturated
  Macronutrient Focus: Protein, healthy fats

- **Eggs**
  Primary Fat: Monounsaturated and saturated
  Macronutrient Focus: Protein, healthy fats

- **Dark Chocolate (70%+ cocoa)**
  Primary Fat: Monounsaturated and saturated
  Macronutrient Focus: Healthy fats, some carbs

- **Coconut (meat, oil, milk)**
  Primary Fat: Plant-based saturated fat
  Macronutrient Focus: Healthy fats

- **Grass-Fed Butter / Ghee**
  Primary Fat: Saturated and omega-3
  Macronutrient Focus: Healthy fats

- **Full-Fat Greek Yogurt**
  Primary Fat: Saturated and monounsaturated
  Macronutrient Focus: Protein, healthy fats

Macros Outline For Your Use

Your macro needs will vary based on your activity level and the type of diet you follow. It's imperative that you consult a qualified dietitian or nutritionist to ensure your targets are safe and appropriate for your goals.

Personal Nutrition Overview

- Ideal Weight: _____; Goal Weight: _____.

- Approximate Calories Per Day: _____

- Meals Per Day: _____

- Calories Per Meal (approx.): _____

Macronutrient Breakdown (Per Meal)

- Protein: _____ grams – *your number one focus!* **Guideline: 0.75–1g** per pound of body weight per day for *most* gym goers; Some suggest eating the number of grams of protein equal to your goal weight, not present weight. *However, it's best to consult a qualified nutritionist or dietitian to determine what's right for you.*

- **Carbohydrates:** _____ **gram**s. *Adjust based on activity level and energy needs*

- **Fats:** _____ **gram**s. *Supports hormones, energy, and satiety*

Additional Nutritional Targets:
- **Fiber** (Daily): 25–50g *Aids digestion and blood sugar control*

- **Sugar** (Daily): <25–50g *Avoid added sugars, especially fructose Check labels:*

sugar shouldn't be one of the first 3 ingredients, limit servings to <10–12g of sugar when possible

- **Sodium**: 1,500–2,000mg/*day*, increase if sweating heavily; *if you have high blood pressure:* <1,500mg **(consult a doctor)**

Diet Notes & Personalization:

There is no one-size-fits-all approach. Some people thrive on low-carb, others on low-fat, so it's important to identify food preferences before building a plan. Meat eaters may benefit from a modified Paleo approach, while fad diets like Keto or Atkins can work in the short term but are rarely sustainable. Regardless of style, the focus should stay on whole foods, limited processed items, consistent protein intake, and steady calorie control for long-term success. When in doubt, seek guidance from a registered dietitian or nutritionist.

Final Thoughts:

- Protein is your priority

- Focus on weekly calorie averages – not daily fluctuations

- Cheat meals are okay – <u>never</u> cheat days

- Build sustainable habits – nutrition is a lifestyle

Nutrient Absorption & Healthy Fats: **Fat helps absorb vitamins A, D, E, and K from vegetables. Without it, you risk wasting key nutrients. Include small amounts of healthy fats like olive oil, butter, or avocado to enhance absorption and support overall health. Avoid empty calories.**

Chapter 15
EFFECTIVE DIETS AND GUIDELINES

Why Do Some Diet Books Fail, While Others Work?

It's not a "special diet" that makes the difference—unless you have a glandular or endocrine disorder.

What truly matters is finding ***an approach that fits you***. Many diets work not because they're extreme, but because they offer a structure people can enjoy and sustain—whether it's by allowing favorite foods or progressing in manageable steps.

Forget the quick fixes and trendy promises. The only diet that will truly work is the one you can live with long-term. Deep down, you already know the kind of eating plan that suits your metabolism, your cravings, and your lifestyle. For some, that might mean fasting for 8–12 hours; for others, especially those with diabetes or hypoglycemia—it means eating more regularly.

Lasting success doesn't come from what someone else swears by—it comes from choosing what's realistic, not what's radical.

KEY POINT: A great way to kick-start your fitness journey is to try **Keto** or **Atkins** short-term. Once you are used to analyzing your daily intake, at the right time, transition to a long-term sustainable meal plan!

Avoid simple carbs, added sugar, and processed foods—anything that spikes insulin; plus, <u>keep calories in Line</u>!. Sustainable meal plans are built around your caloric needs. Every athlete and trainer understands this, including movie stars like Sly, who once said, *"When training for a movie, if my trainer tells me to eat tuna out of the can, I do it!"* – That's the reality for most people—proper calorie intake and macronutrient balance make the difference.

Standardize Your Meals

A higher-protein diet is essential for fat loss while preserving muscle mass, which helps maintain a higher metabolism for long-term success. Focus on losing body fat, not just weight, and ensure you meet your protein needs to support muscle preservation and avoid short-term fixes.

1. **Limiting white flour, white rice, processed food and deli meats, is huge way to begin this journey.**

2. Virtually no soda, sweet tea, fried food, or junk food.

If you need to lose weight, **avoid eating carbs at breakfast,** wait for a few hours, or consider doing so at lunch instead. If you train in the morning then after you exercise would be a good time for your first allowed amount, because they replenish glycogen stores in the muscles; the stored form of glucose that muscles use for energy during workouts.

"At the end of the day, weight loss depends on maintaining a calorie deficit. However, delaying carbohydrate intake—such as skipping them at breakfast and saving them for lunch or post-exercise—can enhance fat burning and improve metabolic efficiency. If you train in the morning, consuming ~1–1.5☐g carbohydrates per kg of bodyweight within ~30☐minutes after your workout (**ideally with some protein**) supports rapid glycogen replenishment and recovery. While individual needs vary, this strategy offers a refined, science-based framework to help your readers reach their goals."

6 Small Meals: This approach helped my first client, Amanda, lose 80lbs. within 1 year even without exercise. While this can lead to a reduction in body fat, it's important to note that muscle tone and overall strength are *best achieved when resistance training is part of the plan.* **What it is:** Eating smaller, more frequent meals helps maintain energy throughout the day, prevents extreme hunger, and supports healthy portion control. It's not about perfection—it's about consistency and building habits that last. See below; 6-small meals.

Pros: Stable energy levels, Reduced cravings, Better portion control, Improved digestion, Consistent blood sugar

Cons: Time-consuming, May lead to overeating for some but not for others, Not ideal for everyone, Social challenges.

A Relationship with Food: We all need to have a good relationship with food—not something we fear or hate, but something we respect and enjoy. After all, food is good. I'm glad we have it. And like most people, I've battled over the years to eat healthy more often than not. What I've found is simple: **balance wins.**

"I eat what I enjoy—if it's good for me. And I'll still eat what I don't love—if it nourishes me. I avoid what harms my body, except on rare occasions. That's not restriction. That's discipline guided by grace."

Deprivation doesn't work. I read about an elite athlete who eats a piece of 86% dark chocolate every day. Why? Because he loves it. And he fits it into his calorie count. That's balance. That's grace. You don't have to earn it. You don't have to punish yourself for it. But you do have to be honest with yourself.

Enjoy the things you love *within reason*. Just don't use that as an excuse to overdo what you know you shouldn't.

We all know the truth: an apple is healthier than a candy bar. But that doesn't make a Snickers bar evil. Enjoy one on occasion—guilt-free—and move on.

View food as fuel. You wouldn't pour Coca-Cola into a gas tank, or put the wrong grade of fuel into a high-performance engine. But people take better care of their cars than they do their own bodies.

Your body is **the only place you have to live in**. Treat it with love. Eat well, not because you hate your body, but because you *love it*. Move your body, not because you're punishing it, but because you want it to run like the powerful, capable machine it was meant to be.

Give yourself grace. Feed your body with intention. Nourish your temple—because it's the only one you've got.

Low-Carb Works—But Not Forever

When you're facing a serious weight loss challenge, one strategy I highly recommend is starting with a low-carb diet. Diets like keto or Atkins can be extremely effective in the short term — especially Atkins, which is a bit more flexible and easier to follow for most people.

That said, it's important to be realistic. Very low-carb diets can be tough to sustain. While you'll find plenty of articles debating the long-term safety of these diets, the truth is, your body **does** need carbohydrates — especially if you're burning energy through exercise, working a physically demanding job, or staying active throughout the day.

Carbs fuel your workouts, replenish glycogen stores in your muscles, and support cognitive function. The amount you need depends on your activity level:

- Are you running or doing high-intensity training?

- Do you work outdoors or have a job that requires movement all day?

If so, eliminating carbs completely isn't ideal — but lowering your intake temporarily can kickstart your metabolism and get you mentally and emotionally aligned with your weight loss goals.

> **Here's what I recommend:**
> - Start with a low-carb approach (either keto or Atkins) for **about six weeks.**
>
> - Monitor how your body responds, and adjust if needed.
>
> - After that, transition into a more balanced, sustainable plan like the **Mediterranean diet** or one of the other healthy options listed in this book.
>
> Everyone's different. I can't personalize this advice for each reader, so I encourage you to consult a knowledgeable personal trainer or registered nutritionist — and be selective. Not all are created equal.
>
> A low-carb diet can be a powerful tool, especially at the start. Use it wisely, and then build a long-term strategy that fits your life.

Grace-Based Eating Principles

Grace-based eating is an approach to food and nutrition rooted in **self-compassion**, **balance**, and **mindfulness**—not guilt, restriction, or rigid rules. It integrates the values of grace—**kindness, forgiveness, and understanding**—into everyday eating habits.

1. Freedom from Dieting Rules

- Let go of strict food rules or labeling foods as "good" or "bad."

- **Focus on nourishment, satisfaction, and sustainability—not deprivation.**

2. Mindful Eating

- **Tune in to hunger and fullness cues.**

- Eat with intention and presence—away from distractions—savoring each bite.

3. Self-Compassion

- Accept moments of indulgence or overeating without shame.

- Replace self-judgment with curiosity and gentle understanding.

4. Balanced Nutrition

- Enjoy a wide variety of foods that support energy, nourishment, and pleasure.

- Understand that most foods can belong in a healthy lifestyle when eaten **with balance**.

5. Emotional Awareness

- Recognize emotional eating as a signal, not a failure.

- Gently explore what's underneath the craving and discover non-food tools for stress, sadness, or boredom.

6. Focus on Well-Being, Not Perfection

- Celebrate progress, not perfection.

- Remember: true health includes the body *and* the heart—physical, mental, and emotional.

Benefits of Grace-Based Eating

- Reduced guilt and anxiety around food

- Improved relationship with eating and body image

- More sustainable health habits

- Increased awareness and emotional resilience

- Greater joy and freedom at the table and beyond

6 Small Meals – 1 Day Example

Meal 1: Greek yogurt with berries and a sprinkle of granola
Meal 2: Boiled egg with cucumber and tomato slices
Meal 3: Turkey lettuce wraps with avocado and shredded carrots
Meal 4: Apple with almond butter
Meal 5: Grilled chicken with roasted vegetables and cauliflower rice
Meal 6: Cottage cheese with blueberries or walnuts

Balanced Diet

What it is: A well-rounded approach including all food groups in appropriate portions.
Pros: Flexible, sustainable, meets nutrient needs.
Cons: Can lack structure; may not lead to fast weight loss.

Mediterranean Diet

What it is: A heart-healthy, anti-inflammatory way of eating inspired by traditional cuisines of southern Europe. It emphasizes whole foods, healthy fats, and balanced portions that promote longevity and wellness.
Pros: Heart-healthy • Supports sustainable fat loss • Rich in fiber and antioxidants • Easy to follow

Cons: Requires regular cooking • Portion control still matters • Not ideal for strict low-carb needs

Zone Diet

What it is: A 40% carb, 30% protein, 30% fat plan to balance hormones and blood sugar.
Pros: Encourages portion control and balanced meals.
Cons: Requires measuring; may be confusing to maintain.

Palm Beach Diet

What it is: A heart-healthy, low-glycemic plan emphasizing lean protein, healthy fats, and good carbs.
Pros: Balanced and nutrient-rich; supports heart health.
Cons: May require label reading and planning; slower weight loss.

Dukan Diet

What it is: A high-protein, very low-carb diet with strict phases.
Pros: Rapid weight loss, appetite control.
Cons: Restrictive, low in nutrients, hard to sustain long-term.

Paleo Diet

What it is: Eat like early humans—meats, veggies, fruits, various nuts; no grains, dairy, or legumes.
Pros: Whole-food focused; reduces processed foods.
Cons: Restrictive; excludes food groups with proven benefits.

DASH Diet

What it is: Developed to lower blood pressure using low-sodium, high-nutrient foods.
Pros: Proven to lower BP and cholesterol; promotes overall health.
Cons: May require effort to reduce salt and processed foods; slower weight loss.

Keto Diet

What it is: High-fat, very low-carb diet to shift the body into fat-burning ketosis.
Pros: Fast weight loss; reduces hunger for some.
Cons: Hard to maintain; may cause side effects; not ideal for all health conditions.

Intermittent Fasting (IF)

What it is: Eat within specific time windows (like 16:8 or 5:2); focuses on *when* you eat, not *what*.
Pros: Can simplify eating, improve insulin sensitivity.
Cons: May cause fatigue or irritability; not for those with blood sugar issues without guidance.

Intermittent fasting is a favorite. It was common in past decades when families ate structured meals: breakfast at 6 AM, lunch at noon, and dinner between 5 and 7 PM—without frequent snacking, so roughly 12 hours between breakfast and dinner. This is how I ate as a youth. Everyone was more active and ate fewer processed foods, contributing to lower obesity rates.

> "Genetics and metabolism play a significant role in shaping body composition. People from different backgrounds may naturally have varying body frames and predispositions. For instance, some populations tend to have more compact builds, while others may have larger skeletal structures due to genetic and environmental factors. Body types—ectomorph, mesomorph, and endomorph—also influence how individuals store fat and build muscle. Even among elite athletes, noticeable differences in muscle tone and physique can occur, sometimes even within the same family."

Most importantly, **eat whole foods as close as possible to how God made them. If man touched them, he likely messed them up.** Avoid processed foods and sugars as much as possible. Eating whole, unprocessed foods is the healthiest and most sustainable way to nourish your body for life.

Atkins Diet

What it is: A low-carb, higher-protein diet that promotes fat burning by limiting carbohydrates.
Pros: Rapid initial weight loss, reduced appetite, gradual carb reintroduction.
Cons: Early fatigue or "keto flu," limited fruits and grains, hard to sustain long-term.
Compared to Keto: Atkins allows carbs to increase over time, while keto stays strictly low-carb and higher in fat.

Pre-Workout Meals

Proper nutrition before workouts enhances performance, provides energy, and improves recovery. The ideal pre-workout meal depends on factors like workout type, intensity, timing, and personal tolerance. This guide offers science-backed tips for optimizing pre-workout nutrition.

Key Factors to Consider

Type of Exercise:

- **Cardio (e.g., running, sprints):** Focus on carbohydrates for energy and protein for muscle preservation.

- **Weightlifting (light or heavy):** Prioritize protein and moderate carbohydrates to sustain energy and facilitate muscle repair.

- **Duration:** Longer workouts require more sustained energy sources, such as complex carbohydrates.

- **Individual Variability:** Digestive tolerance, age, gender, and fitness level all influence the best meal plan.

Timing of Pre-Workout Meals:

- Allows adequate digestion and prevents discomfort during exercise.

- Opt for easily digestible foods if closer to the workout (e.g., smoothies or protein shakes).

- If fasting, ensure proper hydration and consider eating a balanced meal post-workout.

I don't believe in many modern pre-workout energy drinks. A proper diet can help you achieve fitness and maintain energy, especially when carb-loading before a long event. Food is a reliable energy source. Energy drinks offer short-term boosts but aren't advisable except on rare occasions. Stick with food; it has always been effective. Before energy drinks, athletes relied on balanced meals timed to coincide with events, and this approach still works today.

Nutrition For Performance

Afternoon/Evening Workouts: Adjust meals based on your day's food intake and workout intensity.

1. The Purpose of Pre-Workout Nutrition

The goal of pre-workout nutrition is simple: fuel your body for maximum performance. The right combination of nutrients can increase stamina, support mental clarity, reduce fatigue, and minimize soreness. Whether training for strength, endurance, or fat loss, eating smart before a workout sets the tone for results.

2. Understanding Macronutrients

Carbohydrates

Why: Primary energy source—especially for high-intensity workouts.

Examples:

Oatmeal with raisins and walnuts (a personal favorite)

Whole-grain toast with almond butter

Bananas with almond butter (another favorite)

Wild, brown, or basmati rice (another go-to)

Protein: *Why:* Essential for muscle repair and recovery, especially after resistance training.

Examples:

- Protein shakes
- Eggs
- Protein bars

Fats — why: Slower-digesting energy, better for lower-intensity or endurance training.
Examples:
- Avocados
- Almond butter
- Chia seeds

3. Sample Pre-Workout Meals
45–90 Minutes Before Workout

Protein shake with a banana (add strawberries, chia seeds, or flaxseed for fiber)

Whole-grain toast with almond butter and a drizzle of honey

Small serving of oatmeal with raisins and walnuts

Banana with almond or peanut butter (a longtime favorite)

1–2 Hours Before Workout

Grilled chicken with rice and steamed vegetables

Avocado toast with eggs

Smoothie with berries, spinach, almond milk, and protein powder

Yogurt with fruit

Peanut butter, banana, and whole-grain toast

Protein smoothie

Cottage cheese with fruit

Egg wrap

4. Special Considerations

Fasting: Some prefer training fasted, especially in the morning. That can work, but post-workout protein is critical for recovery and growth.

Weight Loss Goals: Skip high-sugar, fruit-heavy smoothies. Choose lower-calorie, nutrient-dense options that energize without overshooting goals.

Digestive Sensitivities: If prone to bloating or discomfort, choose lighter or liquid meals like smoothies and shakes closer to training.

5. Hydration

Hydration matters before, during, and after your workout.

Sip water throughout the day, not just pre-training

Add a pinch of Himalayan salt for short, high-intensity efforts

Use non-sugar electrolyte drinks if sweating heavily or training in heat

6. Post-Workout Nutrition

Refuel within 1–2 hours post-workout. Focus on protein for muscle repair and moderate carbs for energy replenishment.

Grilled chicken with quinoa

Protein smoothie with berries

Scrambled eggs with whole-grain toast

Greek yogurt with fruit and chia seeds

Conclusion: Pre- and post-workout meals aren't just food—they fuel your purpose. Listen to your body, eat with intention, adjust for your goals. Fuel smart, train stronger, grow into the best version of yourself.

Creatine & BCAAs

CREATINE – Boosts strength & power: improves performance:

- Increases muscle mass: promotes growth
- Enhances cognition: supports memory and thinking
- Aids recovery: reduces muscle damage and inflammation
- Supports overall health: benefits bone, heart, insulin sensitivity
- Hydration: drink ~½ your body weight in ounces daily (consult your provider)
- **Who it's for:** Anyone focused on strength, fitness, or well-being. Not just for men—women also benefit.

Benefits for Women – Strength & Lean Muscle Tone:
- Boosts strength and endurance
- Supports lean muscle growth without bulk
- Improves body composition for a more toned look

Enhanced Exercise Performance:

- Increases energy for high-intensity work
- Delays fatigue for more reps/longer sessions
- Improves training capacity and consistency

Faster Recovery:
- Reduces soreness
- Speeds recovery between sessions

Brain & Cognitive Support:
- May improve memory, focus, clarity
- Reduces brain fog during stress

Bone Health:
- Helps maintain bone density
- May reduce risk of osteoporosis

Hydration & Muscle Definition:
- Improves muscle hydration and fullness

Reduces cramps:
- Supports joint function and nutrient delivery

Hormonal Balance & Mood:
- Helps reduce stress-related fatigue
- May support mood stability during intense training or hormonal shifts

Weight & Appearance: A small increase in weight may occur from water in muscle cells. This is not fat—muscles look fuller, more defined.
- **Usage:** Safe at 3–5 g daily. Take pre- or post-workout, or with a meal.

References:

Kreider RB et al. *International Society of Sports Nutrition position stand: safety and efficacy of creatine supplementation in exercise, sport, and medicine.* J Int Soc Sports Nutr (2017).

Forbes SC et al. *Effects of creatine supplementation on performance and training adaptations.* Mol Cell Biochem (2021).

BCAAs (Branched-Chain Amino Acids):

- Boost muscle growth & recovery: stimulate protein synthesis, reduce soreness

- Enhance exercise performance: reduce fatigue, improve endurance

- Support weight management: aid fat burning, appetite control

- Strengthen immune system: support function during training

- Prevent muscle loss: protect lean mass during calorie restriction

- Regulate blood sugar: improve uptake and insulin sensitivity

Dosage: 5–20 g/day around workouts
Safety: Generally safe, consult a healthcare professional

References (succinct):

Wolfe RR. *Branched-chain amino acids and muscle protein synthesis in humans: myth or reality?* J Int Soc Sports Nutr (2017).

Shimomura Y et al. *Branched-chain amino acid supplementation before squat exercise and delayed-onset muscle soreness.* Int J Sport Nutr Exerc Metab (2010).

GOOD, NOT SO GOOD

Basic Foods You Can Eat Often

Based on guidance from the Mayo Clinic, Harvard School of Public Health, and the American Heart Association.

Eating healthy fats with vegetables helps your body absorb key nutrients—vitamins A, D, E, and K, along with antioxidants like carotenoids found in carrots, spinach, and bell peppers. These nutrients need fat for proper digestion and absorption. In short: adding a little olive oil, avocado, or butter (grass-fed or other) unlocks their full nutritional power and turns a good meal into a great one.

Whole, nutrient-dense, anti-inflammatory:

- **Leafy greens** – spinach, kale, arugula, Swiss chard
- **Cruciferous vegetables** – broccoli, cauliflower, Brussels sprouts
- **Berries** – blueberries, strawberries, raspberries (high in antioxidants, low in sugar)
- **Fatty fish** – salmon, mackerel, sardines (rich in omega-3s)
- **Nuts & seeds** – almonds, walnuts, pecans, chia, flax (healthy fats and fiber)
- **Legumes** – lentils, black beans, chickpeas
- **Whole grains** – oats, quinoa, brown rice (*limit if insulin resistant*)
- **Olive oil – extra virgin, cold-pressed, unrefined (a natural anti-inflammatory).**
- **Avocados** – high in monounsaturated fats and potassium
- **Water & herbal teas** – support hydration, digestion, and metabolism

Eat These For Vitamin D

Why Vitamin D Matters:

- Supports bone and teeth strength

- Boosts immune defense

- Helps regulate mood and mental health (low levels linked to depression)

- Improves muscle function

- May reduce inflammation

- May play a role in weight management and metabolism

Top Food Sources:
- Salmon (wild-caught preferred)

- Mackerel

- Sardines

- Tuna (canned in oil)

- Cod liver oil (1 tsp provides more than a day's requirement)

- Egg yolks

- Beef liver

- Fortified milk (dairy or plant-based)

- Fortified cereals

- Fortified orange juice

- UV-exposed mushrooms (e.g., maitake, portobello)

Other Key Sources:
- Sunlight (natural and free)

- Supplements (Vitamin D3 is preferred for absorption)

Foods You Can Eat in Moderation

Okay occasionally or in small portions
- **Lean red meat** – grass-fed beef, lamb (*1–2x/week max*)

- **Poultry** – chicken or turkey without skin

- **Eggs** – For most healthy people, **two to three per day is safe**.

- **Starchy vegetables** – sweet potatoes, corn, peas

- **Whole wheat bread or pasta** – choose **100% whole grain** and eat small portions

Important Note on Grains:
- **Whole Grain**: Contains **bran, germ, and endosperm** – must be **dense**, not soft. Real whole grain bread should be so hearty that, as mentioned elsewhere in this book, *if you threw it at me, it would hurt.*

- **Refined Grain**: The **bran and germ are removed**, leaving only the **starchy endosperm**. It's often **pulverized** into fine flour, making the result less nutritious, higher on the glycemic index, and stripped of fiber.

Other moderation foods:
- **Dark chocolate** – 70%+ cocoa, 1 oz per serving

- **Natural cheeses** – small portions, avoid processed types

- **Coffee** – up to 2 cups per day (black or lightly sweetened)

- **Wine** – If you drink, limit to **1 glass per day** at most, and only with your doctor's approval. Some studies once suggested wine protects the heart, but newer research shows **any alcohol increases health risks**, including cancer. Bottom line: **wine is not necessary for health**. If you don't drink, there's no reason to start.

- **Protein bars or powders** – choose low sugar, minimally processed options

Eggs - Mega Nutrition

Eggs are packed with essential nutrients, making them one of the most nutrient-dense foods. Here's a breakdown of the key nutrients found in an egg and how the body absorbs them:

Nutrients in an Egg (Per Large Egg - ~50g)
Macronutrients:
- **Protein** (4-6g) – High-quality complete protein with all essential amino acids.
- **Fats** (3-5g) – Includes healthy monounsaturated and polyunsaturated fats.
- **Carbohydrates** (<0.5g) – Very minimal.
- **Calories** (70-90 kcal) – Provides sustained energy.

Vitamins:
- **Vitamin A** – Supports vision, immune health, and skin.
- **Vitamin D** – Essential for calcium absorption and bone health.
- **Vitamin E** – Acts as an antioxidant, protecting cells.
- **Vitamin K** – Helps with blood clotting and bone health.
- **B Vitamins (B2, B5, B6, B12, Folate, Biotin, Choline)** – Aid in energy production, brain function, and red blood cell formation.

Minerals:
- **Iron** – Essential for oxygen transport in the blood.
- **Zinc** – Supports immunity and wound healing.
- **Phosphorus** – Important for bones and teeth.

- **Selenium** – A powerful antioxidant.

- **Iodine** – Necessary for thyroid function.

Other Important Compounds:
- **Choline** – Critical for brain and nervous system health.

- **Lutein & Zeaxanthin** – Protects eye health by reducing the risk of macular degeneration.

How the Body Absorbs Nutrients from Eggs
- **Digestion Starts in the Stomach** – Enzymes and stomach acid break down proteins into amino acids.

- **Small Intestine Absorption** – *Nutrients are absorbed into the bloodstream:*

- **Proteins** → Absorbs as amino acids, used for muscle repair and enzyme production.

- **Fats** → Broken into fatty acids and absorbed through the lymphatic system.

- **Fat-Soluble Vitamins (A, D, E, K)** → Absorbs fats and requires bile from the liver.

- **Water-Soluble Vitamins (B, Choline, Folate)** → Directly absorbed into the bloodstream.

- **Minerals (Iron, Zinc, etc.)** → Transported through special carriers for cell use.

- **Liver Processing** – Nutrients are sent to the liver for metabolism and storage.

- **Cell Utilization** – Nutrients are distributed throughout the body for energy, cell repair, and overall function.

Eggs are especially bioavailable, meaning the body efficiently absorbs and uses nutrients. Eating eggs with a source of healthy fat (like avocado) can further enhance the absorption of fat-soluble vitamins.

> Cooking eggs can cause a slight reduction in certain nutrients, particularly heat-sensitive ones like B-complex vitamins (such as B6 and folate), vitamin A, and antioxidants like lutein and zeaxanthin. **Scrambling eggs over high heat or for prolonged periods** may result in *slightly* greater nutrient loss due to increased exposure to heat and oxygen. However, these losses are minimal, and **eggs remain one of the most nutrient-dense foods available. Poached or soft-boiled eggs retain the highest levels of nutrients**, followed by hard-boiled and gently scrambled eggs. Regardless of the method, eggs consistently provide high-quality protein, essential fats, and a wide range of vitamins and minerals.

Foods to Never Eat (or Avoid as Much as Possible)

(Heavily processed, inflammatory, or linked to chronic disease)

- **Processed meats** – bacon, sausage, hot dogs, deli meats (*high in nitrates and sodium*)

- **Sugary beverages** – soda, energy drinks, sweetened teas

- **Refined carbs** – white bread, pastries, doughnuts, white rice

- **Trans fats** – margarine, some baked goods, fried foods

- **Highly processed snacks** – chips, snack cakes, chemical-laden crackers

- **Artificial sweeteners** – especially aspartame, saccharin (*may disrupt gut microbiome*)

- **Fried fast food** – burgers, fries, chicken nuggets (*high in acrylamides and trans fats*)

- **Sugary cereals** – even those labeled "whole grain"

- **Canned soups & frozen dinners** – often very high in sodium and preservatives

- **Excess alcohol** – chronic overuse is linked to cancer, liver damage, and heart disease.

Ultra-Processed Foods

Emerging research increasingly links ultra-processed foods (UPFs) with poor mental health outcomes. These foods—high in added sugars, refined grains, artificial additives, and unhealthy fats—are designed for convenience, taste, and long shelf life, but often lack nutritional value.

Studies have found a strong association between high **UPF consumption and increased risks of depression, anxiety, and cognitive decline**. One proposed mechanism is chronic inflammation: UPFs can disrupt gut microbiota and trigger low-grade systemic inflammation, which is closely connected to brain health and mood regulation. Nutrient deficiencies are also a factor—UPFs tend to displace whole foods rich in vitamins, minerals, and omega-3s, which support neurotransmitter function and emotional balance.

Another contributing factor is blood sugar instability. Many UPFs cause rapid spikes and crashes in glucose levels, leading to irritability, fatigue, and mood swings. Over time, this can affect hormonal and neurological balance, compounding mental health challenges.

Reducing UPFs and replacing them with nutrient-dense whole foods—such as fruits, vegetables, legumes, whole grains, lean proteins, and healthy fats—has been shown to improve mood, reduce depressive symptoms, and enhance overall mental well-being. **The Mediterranean diet,** for example, is frequently cited for its protective effects against depression and anxiety.

> **While UPFs may be hard to avoid completely, increasing awareness and gradually shifting toward whole-food-based eating is a powerful strategy for supporting both body and mind.**

A 2022 meta-analysis of observational studies found that higher ultra-processed food consumption was associated with about **1.44 times the odds** of reporting depressive symptoms and **1.48 times the odds** of reporting anxiety symptoms (higher vs lower intake). The analysis was dominated by cross-sectional data, so it reflects association, not proof of causation.

A 2022 cohort study published in *JAMA Neurology* followed 10,775 adults for a median of eight years. Participants with higher intakes of ultraprocessed foods showed about a 28% faster rate of global cognitive decline and a 25% faster decline in executive function compared with those with the lowest intakes. The study was observational, so it demonstrates association rather than causation.

In the ELSA-Brasil cohort (8,160 participants, ~9 years follow-up), higher ultra-processed food intake (highest vs lowest quintile) was associated with greater declines in executive function and memory performance, though no significant link was found for verbal fluency.

Insulin Issues

Some individuals face insulin issues, where excess sugar in the bloodstream is not efficiently stored or utilized. When your body cannot properly regulate blood sugar, it often results in energy crashes, cravings, and potential long-term health problems.

One of the most effective ways to support healthy blood sugar levels is to **increase muscle mass. Your muscles serve as a storage site for glycogen, the form of glucose your body uses for energy.** The more muscle you have, the more effectively your body can store and utilize carbohydrates, providing steady, lasting energy for your workouts and daily activities.

<u>Heavily processed foods</u> **are engineered to be highly palatable, often leading to overeating**. They are designed to trigger cravings, making it easy to consume excessive calories without realizing it. These foods are usually low in fiber, protein, and healthy fats—the nutrients that help regulate appetite and support metabolism. By concentrating on whole, nutrient-dense foods, such as lean proteins, healthy fats, complex carbohydrates, and plenty of vegetables, you'll naturally feel more satisfied while nourishing your body for optimal performance.

A key mindset shift is to view food as fuel rather than something to restrict. When you prioritize whole foods, eating no longer feels like a restrictive "four-letter word" diet—it becomes a sustainable way of life. **Instead of focusing on what you cannot**

have, focus on what you can, adding more fresh produce, protein-rich meals, and high-fiber foods that keep you full and energized.

Additionally, remember that **one pound of fat equals approximately 3,500 calories.** The average person who eats a diet high in processed foods often consumes hundreds of extra calories each week without even realizing it. These extra calories accumulate over time, making weight management more challenging. Conversely, when you fuel your body with whole food, you're not just managing your weight but enhancing your metabolism, energy levels, and overall well-being.

Consistency is crucial. Small, sustainable changes—like choosing whole grains over refined ones, drinking water instead of sugary drinks, and ensuring adequate protein in meals—can have a significant impact over time. Your body thrives on quality nutrition, and by consistently making better choices, you set yourself up for lifelong success.

Harmful Effects of Sugar

How the Sugar Industry Shaped Modern Health Problems — In My Opinion

Decades ago, the sugar industry funded research that minimized sugar's risks and shifted blame for heart disease to saturated fat. Archival documents from the 1960s show the Sugar Research Foundation influenced Harvard publications that shaped dietary guidelines for decades. This history doesn't make saturated fat harmless, but it explains why sugar's role in chronic disease was overlooked for so long.

More recent studies are clearer: sugar in whole foods acts differently in the body than sugar in liquids. Large analyses show sugar-sweetened beverages (soda, sweet tea, sports drinks, even fruit juice) raise the risk of type 2 diabetes, cardiovascular disease, and hypertension. Each 12-oz daily serving of soda raises diabetes risk by about 25%. Even an 8-oz serving of fruit juice can raise risk by 5%. In contrast, sugar in whole fruits is absorbed slowly because of fiber, water, and nutrients, blunting blood sugar spikes.

Added fructose from processed foods and drinks can promote fat buildup in the liver, contributing to nonalcoholic fatty liver disease (NAFLD). Fructose in fruit rarely has this effect. High intakes of added sugar are also linked to higher triglycerides, lower HDL cholesterol, and poorer cardiometabolic health. Both sugary and artificially sweetened beverages have been associated with higher blood pressure in pooled studies, though causality is less clear for artificial sweeteners.

The effects extend beyond physical health. Observational studies link high sugar intake with greater risk of depression, anxiety, and mood swings, possibly through inflammation and unstable blood sugar. Rapidly absorbed sugars also stimulate brain reward pathways, reinforcing cravings and habit loops. At the cellular level, excess sugar drives glycation, damaging collagen and elastin and potentially accelerating skin aging.

The American Heart Association advises limiting added sugar to no more than 6% of daily calories—about 25 g (6 teaspoons) for women and 36 g (9 teaspoons) for men. Reducing liquid sugar intake is the single most effective step for metabolic health.

Practical strategies include:

- Swap sweets for whole fruit or a small piece of dark chocolate

- Cut back gradually to reduce cravings

- Pair carbs with protein and fiber to stabilize blood sugar

- Stay hydrated to avoid mistaking thirst for hunger

- Read labels for hidden sugars (dextrose, maltose, corn syrup)

- Stay active, since exercise improves insulin sensitivity and appetite control

CARBS, FAT, FIBER

Nutrition isn't just about counting calories—it's about making smart choices that support your metabolism, energy, and long-term health. Knowing which carbohydrates and fats to avoid, and which fiber-rich foods to embrace, can help reduce inflammation, support mental health, and aidin weight management.

Many processed diet foods are sold as "low-fat" or "low-carb," yet they're often packed with added sugars or unhealthy fats. This mix can trigger insulin spikes, promote fat storage, and drive cravings that derail progress.

Carbohydrates

Good - Complex and Nutrient-Dense: These digest slowly, provide steady energy, and are rich in fiber, vitamins, and minerals.

Whole Grains:
- Oats
- Quinoa
- Brown rice – Basmati (my favorite)
- Farro
- Barley
- Buckwheat
- Bulgur wheat
- Millet
- Whole wheat pasta
- Sprouted grain bread (e.g., Ezekiel)

Starchy Vegetables:
- Sweet potatoes
- Butternut squash
- Pumpkin
- Beets
- Parsnips
- Turnips

Legumes:
- Lentils

- Chickpeas
- Black beans
- Kidney beans
- Navy beans
- Edamame
- Green peas

Fruits: Nutrient-Dense, Natural Energy

Fruit is a fantastic source of fiber, antioxidants, vitamins, and hydration. However, some fruits are part of the "Dirty Dozen" list, which means they tend to contain higher pesticide levels when conventionally grown. When possible, choose organic or wash thoroughly, especially for those marked accordingly.

- **Apples** – High in fiber and antioxidants. (*Dirty Dozen – buy organic or wash well*)

- **Berries** (blueberries, raspberries, strawberries, blackberries) – Rich in antioxidants and vitamin C. (*Dirty Dozen – especially strawberries*)

- **Bananas** – Great source of potassium and easy on the digestive system. Less ripe bananas have lower sugar content.

- **Oranges** – Loaded with vitamin C and hydration. Peel protects against pesticide exposure.

- **Pears** – High in fiber and water content. (*Dirty Dozen – wash well or buy organic*)

- **Plums** – Support digestion and provide antioxidants.

- **Grapefruit** – Boosts immunity and may support fat metabolism (check for medication interactions).

- **Kiwi** – High in vitamin C and fiber, supports digestion.

- **Pineapple** – Aids digestion with natural enzymes.

- **Pomegranate** – Packed with antioxidants, heart-healthy compounds.

- **Figs** – High in fiber and natural sugars. Best in moderation.

- **Dates** – Nutrient-dense and energizing, but high in sugar. Use sparingly.

- **Cherries** – Anti-inflammatory and antioxidant-rich. (*Dirty Dozen – wash thoroughly*)

- **Avocados** – Technically a fruit; high in healthy fats and low in sugar. Not on the Dirty Dozen.

- **Olives** – Another fatty fruit, great for heart health. Low pesticide risk.

Vegetables:
- Carrots
- Broccoli
- Brussels sprouts
- Cauliflower
- Zucchini
- Spinach
- Kale
- Swiss chard

Bad Carbohydrates – (Refined and Highly Processed)
These are typically low in fiber and nutrients and spike blood sugar levels.
<u>Refined Grains</u>
- White bread
- White rice
- Regular pasta (not whole grain)

- Baked goods (cakes, cookies, pastries)
- Pancakes and waffles made with white flour
- Crackers made with refined flour

<u>Sugary Foods</u>
- Candy
- Soda
- Sugary cereals
- Energy drinks
- Ice cream
- Sweetened yogurt
- Syrups and jams with added sugar
- Packaged granola bars with added sugar

<u>Fast Food and Processed Snacks</u>
- French fries
- Potato chips
- Nachos
- Fried dough
- Microwave popcorn with additives
- Fast food burgers with white buns

Fats

Healthy: These support brain health, hormones, heart function, and energy balance.

Monounsaturated Fats

- Olive oil

- Avocados

6 Healthiest Nuts

Key Vitamin Highlights

- **Almonds:** Vitamin E, Riboflavin

- **Pistachios:** Vitamin B6, Thiamin

- **Walnuts:** Primarily minerals and omega-3s (no dominant vitamins)

- **Cashews:** Vitamin K, Vitamin B6

- **Macadamias:** Thiamin

- **Pecans:** Thiamin

Polyunsaturated Fats

- Salmon

- Sardines

- Mackerel

- Trout

- Chia seeds

- Flaxseeds

- Hemp seeds

- Walnuts

- Pumpkin seeds

- Sunflower seeds (cold-pressed)

Other Healthy Fat Sources

- Coconut (in moderation)
- Dark chocolate (70% or higher cacao)
- Whole eggs
- Natural nut butters (no added sugar or hydrogenated oils)

Bad Fats (Unhealthy or Inflammatory)

These contribute to inflammation, poor heart health, and metabolic dysfunction.

Trans Fats (Avoid Completely)

- Hydrogenated oils
- Margarine
- Packaged baked goods with trans fats
- Some microwave popcorns
- Non-dairy creamers
- Some frozen pizzas and processed snacks

Excessive Omega-6 Vegetable Oils (Especially When Heated)

- Corn oil
- Soybean oil
- Cottonseed oil
- Safflower oil
- Refined sunflower oil
- Refined canola oil

Deep-Fried and Fast Foods

- French fries

- Fried chicken
- Donuts
- Onion rings
- Deep-fried snacks

Fiber

Gut-Healthy Sources: Fiber aids digestion, nourishes beneficial bacteria, and maintains gut balance. While plant proteins may lack certain essential amino acids, research shows that vegans can build comparable muscle mass with adequate total protein. Fiber also supports muscle growth by enhancing gut health, insulin sensitivity, and recovery.

Insoluble Fiber (Adds Bulk)
- Whole wheat
- Brown rice
- Quinoa *(also soluble)*
- Carrots
- Celery
- Cucumber
- Zucchini
- Nuts and seeds
- Cauliflower
- Green beans

Soluble Fiber (Feeds Gut Bacteria and Aids Digestion)
- Oats
- Quinoa *(also insoluble)*

- Apples
- Bananas
- Beans and lentils
- Psyllium husk
- Flaxseeds
- Chia seeds
- Barley
- Avocados
- Sweet potatoes
- Black mission figs, or most any – moderately high in sugar but also provide water, fiber, and nutrients

Prebiotic-Rich Fiber (Feeds Probiotics in the Gut)
- Asparagus
- Garlic
- Onions
- Leeks
- Dandelion greens
- Jerusalem artichokes

Let's Not Forget... Nutrition isn't just about what you eat—it's also about what you drink and how your body responds.

Alkaline Water & Acidic Foods

Hype, Health, and What Really Matters

In the world of health and fitness, alkaline water and acidic foods often spark heated debates. Some claim alkaline water neutralizes harmful acids in the body, while others warn against the dangers of acidic foods, blaming them for everything from low energy to chronic disease. But what's myth, what's marketing, and what actually helps your body thrive?

Understanding pH Balance in the Body

The pH scale measures how acidic or alkaline a substance is, ranging from 0 (most acidic) to 14 (most alkaline). A pH of 7 is neutral. Your body works hard to keep your blood pH tightly regulated around 7.35–7.45. This is crucial—your cells, enzymes, and organs function properly only within this narrow window.

Contrary to popular belief, the foods and drinks you consume don't drastically change your blood pH. Your lungs and kidneys are constantly adjusting your internal chemistry to maintain that delicate balance.

However, the food you eat can influence the pH of your **urine**, which is why many alkaline diet proponents see changes in their pH strips—but this doesn't mean your blood is changing. Urine pH is more of an indicator of what your body is excreting than what it's absorbing.

Alkaline Water: What It Is and What It Isn't

Alkaline water typically has a pH between 8 and 9.5 and may contain minerals like calcium, potassium, and magnesium. The idea is that drinking alkaline water helps neutralize acidity in the body, potentially improving hydration, reducing acid reflux, and lowering inflammation.

What does science say?

- Some small studies suggest alkaline water may temporarily help with acid reflux and hydration after intense workouts.

- However, there's no strong evidence it changes your body's core pH or provides long-term health benefits.

- For most people, clean, filtered water is just as effective—if not more reliable—than expensive, bottled alkaline water.

If you enjoy the taste of alkaline water or feel it helps you drink more water daily, there's no harm in it. Just don't fall for miracle claims.

Acidic Foods: Not the Villain

Many nutrient-rich foods are technically acidic—think tomatoes, citrus fruits, coffee, lean meats, and eggs. These are not harmful in a balanced diet. In fact, **some of the most alkaline-promoting foods (like lemon juice) are acidic outside the body but have an alkaline-forming effect once metabolized.**

What's more important than a food's pH is how it affects your overall **inflammation, gut health, and nutrient intake**. Acidic junk foods—processed meats, fried snacks, sugary sodas—are unhealthy not because they're acidic, but because they're inflammatory, nutrient-poor, and contribute to metabolic issues.

Balance, Not Extremes

The takeaway? Instead of stressing over alkaline versus acidic labels, focus on eating a diverse, whole-food diet:

- Load up on leafy greens, cruciferous vegetables, berries, legumes, and healthy fats like olive oil and avocado.

- Hydrate with clean water, and add lemon or cucumber slices if you want an alkaline boost.

- Limit heavily processed, high-sodium, and sugar-laden foods that disrupt digestion and energy—not because they're acidic, but because they offer little nutritional value.

Final Thoughts: Alkaline water and acidic foods aren't magic bullets, they're tools and ingredients that play a role in your health—but only as part of the bigger picture. Your body is already doing the hard work of maintaining its balance. Support it by staying hydrated, eating smart, and not getting lost in the hype.

Hydration Check: Urine Color & What It Means

I would be remiss if I didn't mention this simple health marker. What you eat matters, but so does how you hydrate. One of the easiest ways to gauge hydration is by urine color

1. Clear or Transparent: You're likely well-hydrated—but if your urine is always this clear, you may be overhydrating, which can deplete essential electrolytes. It's best to maintain a light straw color instead.

2. Pale Yellow (Light Straw): This is ideal. It means you're well-hydrated and your body is functioning optimally in terms of fluid balance.

3. Bright Yellow: Still within the normal range. Could be a sign of vitamin supplements (especially B vitamins), which are water-soluble and excreted through urine.

4. Dark Yellow: You're slightly dehydrated. Consider drinking more water soon. This is a common color first thing in the morning or after exercise.

5. Amber or Honey Colored: This suggests moderate dehydration. Your body is conserving water, and it's time to rehydrate with fluids—preferably water or electrolyte-rich beverages.

6. Orange: Possible dehydration, but could also be due to food dyes, carrots, or certain medications (like rifampin or some laxatives). If it persists, consult a healthcare provider.

7. Pink or Red: May be caused by foods like beets or berries, but it can also indicate blood in the urine (hematuria), which requires medical evaluation.

8. Blue or Green: Uncommon. Can be linked to food coloring, certain medications, or rare medical conditions. If persistent, see a doctor.

9. Brown: Could be due to dehydration or more serious conditions such as liver or kidney disorders. Needs medical attention if persistent.

10. Cloudy or Murky: May indicate urinary tract infections, kidney stones, or other health issues. Often accompanied by a strong odor and should be evaluated by a professional.

Chapter 16
PROTEIN: YOUR TOP PRIORITY

> Everyone's Needs Are Different—Check With Your Healthcare Provider, or a Qualified Dietitian

General recommendation:

For healthy adults, commonly cited protein intake ranges from approximately 0.8 to 1.0 grams per kilogram of body weight per day, depending on age, activity level, and overall health status. This aligns with guidance referenced by the Mayo Clinic and the National Institutes of Health.

> **IMPORTANT MEDICAL CAUTION:** Individuals with chronic kidney disease (CKD), reduced kidney function, elevated serum creatinine, or other diagnosed renal conditions may require lower protein intake. In these cases, higher protein consumption can increase renal workload and may contribute to further decline in kidney function if not medically supervised. Anyone with known kidney disease, abnormal kidney lab values, or a history of renal issues should not increase protein intake without guidance from a physician or registered dietitian. In these

situations, protein intake is a medical decision, not a general fitness recommendation.

Clinical guidelines, including those referenced by the National Kidney Foundation, often recommend protein restriction in later stages of kidney disease, with intake individualized based on:

- stage of kidney disease

- laboratory values such as eGFR, creatinine, and BUN

- overall medical management

FUNDAMENTALS

1. Caloric Balance is Key

The foundation of weight management is **calories in versus calories out**. No matter what dietary approach you follow, your body needs to burn more calories than it consumes to lose weight or consume more than it burns to gain weight. This principle should be at the forefront of your mind when adjusting your diet.

2. Protein's Vital Role

Protein is essential, especially if you exercise regularly and engage in resistance or strength training. When you work your muscles hard, they require protein to repair and grow, preventing muscle breakdown.

3. Balancing Carbs and Fats

When it comes to carbs and fats, there's flexibility depending on your activity level and metabolism. Some days, you may need more carbs (especially on heavy workout days), while on other days, you might want to reduce them. The key is to adjust based on your energy expenditure. However, if you have specific health conditions like diabetes or heart issues, be cautious with high-fat or low-carb diets and consult a healthcare professional before making significant dietary changes.

4. No Magic Diet—Consistency is Key

Various diets have trended, from low-fat diets in the '60s and '70s to low-carb options like keto in the '90s. No single macronutrient causes weight gain; it's the excess of calories that matters. Prioritize protein and balance fat and carbs according to your needs. **Each** diet book has helped many, but others found no help; this illustrates the need for a personalized approach. What works for one person may not work for another.

5. Effort and Discipline are Crucial

Ultimately, no diet will be successful without the right mindset. **Effort, discipline, and consistency** are the most critical elements of fitness success. Showing up with intention, pushing yourself in your workouts, and following a balanced and well-thought-out diet will yield results. *Focus on giving 100% effort, and the results will follow.*

Start Your Day with Protein

Whether you're building strength, managing weight, or just staying energized, for *some* individuals, one of the smartest moves is to begin your day with protein. It curbs cravings, supports muscle recovery, and jumpstarts metabolism. Aim for about 0.75–0.82 grams per pound of body weight daily—up to 1 gram for *some* individuals. <u>**Exact needs vary by goals, diet, and activity, so consult a dietitian for a personalized plan.**</u>

Protein digestion vs. muscle building:

The body can digest and absorb more than 25–30 grams of protein in a single meal; there is no fixed upper limit to protein digestion. That commonly cited number refers to muscle protein synthesis, not digestion. Muscle protein synthesis appears to be maximally stimulated at approximately 20–40 grams per meal, depending on body size, age, and activity level. Protein consumed beyond this amount is still absorbed and used by the body, but **protein is not stored for future use**; excess amino acids are utilized for other physiological functions or oxidized for energy rather than held in reserve.

Why Protein Matters More Than You Think:

- **Keeps you full:** High-protein meals curb hunger better than carb- or fat-heavy ones.

- **Stabilizes blood sugar:** Slows digestion and helps prevent energy crashes.

- **Boosts metabolism:** Whole-food proteins—especially animal-based—have a thermogenic effect, meaning your body burns more calories digesting them.

- **Preserves lean muscle:** Critical for fat loss and long-term body composition.

Practical Tips
- **Start with breakfast:** Eggs, Greek yogurt, or a protein shake can anchor your day.

- **Use lean sources:** Chicken, turkey, fish, eggs, lean beef, and low-fat dairy are excellent choices.

- **Drink it if you can't eat it:** Protein shakes are a convenient backup when you're short on time or appetite.

The Recommended Dietary Allowance (RDA) for protein represents the minimum intake required to prevent deficiency in the general population. It is intentionally conservative and does not account for higher needs associated with physical activity, aging, recovery, or training.

Many dietary and clinical guidelines recommend higher protein intake for active individuals, older adults, and those engaged in regular resistance or endurance exercise. In practice, protein needs are often estimated using body weight and activity level to better reflect real-world demands while remaining within safe and accepted ranges.

Different dietary approaches use different protein targets, and individual needs can vary based on health status, training volume, and metabolic factors. For this reason, protein recommendations should be viewed as guidelines rather than absolutes.

Individuals with medical conditions affecting protein metabolism or kidney function should consult with a registered dietitian or qualified healthcare professional to determine appropriate intake.

Protein intake is best distributed evenly across meals and adjusted based on goals, body composition, and activity level.

Protein Needs (per pound of body weight):

Sedentary (general health): ~0.36 g/lb

Covers basic maintenance and essential physiological functions.

Lightly active / recreational activity: 0.45–0.55 g/lb

Supports activity demands and recovery.

Endurance athletes: 0.55–0.64 g/lb
Helps prevent muscle breakdown and supports endurance recovery.

Strength training / muscle gain: 0.7–0.85 g/lb
Supports muscle repair, growth, and strength adaptations.

Fat loss / caloric deficit: 0.8–1.0 g/lb
Helps preserve lean mass during reduced calorie intake.

Older adults (65+): 0.55–0.68 g/lb
Supports maintenance of lean mass, strength, and mobility.

Pregnancy / breastfeeding:
Protein needs increase during pregnancy and lactation and should be individualized based on body weight, trimester or lactation stage, and medical guidance.

References:
Institute of Medicine. Dietary Reference Intakes for Protein (2005).
Phillips SM & Van Loon LJC. Journal of Sports Sciences (2011).
Morton RW et al.. British Journal of Sports Medicine (2018).

Thermogenetic Effect of Protein & Weight Management

Protein does more than support muscle—it also increases calorie burn through digestion, known as the **thermic effect of food (TEF)**. Protein has the highest TEF of all macronutrients: about **20–30%** of its calories are used during digestion and processing, compared with **5–10% for carbohydrates** and **0–3% for fats**.

Animal proteins (meat, fish, eggs, dairy) generally have a slightly higher thermic effect than most plant proteins, especially when minimally processed. This doesn't mean plant proteins aren't valuable, but for fat loss and metabolism support, animal sources are usually more metabolically demanding.

Higher protein intake—especially from high-quality sources—can help:

- Boost resting energy expenditure

- Preserve lean muscle during weight loss

- Reduce appetite and cravings

- Improve satiety and blood sugar stability

The benefits depend on **quality, digestibility, and amino acid profile**. For best results, prioritize complete proteins (those with all essential amino acids) and spread intake evenly across the day.

Meal Timing: Eating every 3–4 hours helps maintain steady energy, though needs vary by activity level and dietary approach. Each meal or snack should ideally include lean protein, complex carbs, and water for balance and sustained energy.

References (succinct):

Westerterp KR. *Diet induced thermogenesis.* Nutr Metab (2017).

Halton TL & Hu FB. *The effects of high protein diets on thermogenesis, satiety and weight loss.* J Am Coll Nutr (2004).

Paddon-Jones D et al. *Protein, weight management, and satiety.* Am J Clin Nutr (2008).

Focus on Weekly Balance:

Hydration matters. Aim for approximately **8–9 glasses of water per day**, or roughly **half your body weight in ounces**, adjusting for activity level, environment, and individual health factors. Hydration needs vary, so consult a qualified healthcare provider if you are unsure.

A few higher-calorie days will not derail progress **as long as overall weekly intake remains consistent**. Weekly balance matters more than daily perfection.

Prioritize protein. When protein intake is adequate, overall food choices and calorie control often improve naturally.

Research indicates that increasing protein intake from approximately **15% to 30% of daily calories** can lead to a spontaneous reduction in total energy intake—often by **several hundred calories per day**—without deliberate calorie restriction.

> **For most meal plans or diets, keep it simple: prioritize protein, then balance the rest.**

Buying Fish: Fresh Or Frozen?

My first recommendation is to choose fish that are low on the food chain.
These short-lived, non-predatory fish (such as sardines, anchovies, herring, trout, and smaller salmon) naturally contain rich omega-3s, high-quality protein, and essential trace minerals, but **without the heavy toxin load** found in large predatory species.

Bioaccumulation: The Double-Edged Sword

While all fish contain valuable nutrients, species that *eat other fish*—including tuna, swordfish, king mackerel, and shark—accumulate higher concentrations of mercury and PCBs as they climb the food chain. This process, known as bioaccumulation, makes large predatory fish riskier for frequent consumption. Choosing smaller, shorter-lived fish keeps the nutrients while minimizing toxin exposure.

Why Choose Frozen Fish from Reputable Fisheries Over "Fresh" Market Fish
Frozen fish from reputable fisheries is processed and blast-frozen immediately after being caught, which preserves its freshness, quality, and nutritional value. Many "fresh" fish at markets have actually been out of the water for a week or more before reaching consumers.

Farm-raised fish can be convenient, but quality varies widely. In less-regulated farms, overcrowding can lead to increased waste and the use of antibiotics, which may leave residues if oversight is poor. For this reason, I generally prefer wild-caught fish when possible. While some wild species carry mercury concerns, it's a trade-off that depends on species, size, and diet, not simply whether the fish is wild or farmed.

If you live near the Gulf or the ocean, you can often get excellent product directly from local fishermen. Just remember that boats may stay out for several days, and even with dry ice, the fish can be up to a week old before returning—still a very good choice.

Large commercial fisheries process, fillet, and blast-freeze their catch at temperatures near −30°, locking in freshness at its peak. Also an excellent choice.

I personally prefer Atlantic and Sockeye salmon for their high omega-3 content, with Sockeye being slightly higher. Tuna steaks such as albacore and bluefin are solid second choices.

Many reputable companies ship wild-caught Alaska or Atlantic salmon overnight, packed in dry ice. These fish are often only a few days old by the time they reach your home.

Buying Smart

At many delis and seafood counters, fish advertised as "fresh" is often previously frozen and thawed for display. Always ask. Mislabeling is common.

When buying whole fish, look for bright red gills, firm flesh, and a clean ocean smell. Grey gills, mushy texture, or a strong fishy odor indicate deterioration.

My background includes 18 years as a beef and seafood purchaser, and these principles have held true everywhere I've worked.

10 Signs You're Not Eating Enough Protein

1. Constant Hunger: Protein helps keep you full. Without enough protein, you might feel hungry soon after meals.

2. Muscle Loss: Protein is crucial for muscle maintenance. Deficiency can lead to muscle wasting and decreased strength.

3. Weak Immune System: Protein is essential for building and repairing tissues, including immune cells. A lack of protein can make you more susceptible to illnesses.

4. Hair, Skin, and Nail Problems: Protein is a key component of hair, skin, and nails. Deficiency can lead to brittle nails, hair loss, and skin problems.

5. Fatigue and Weakness: Without enough protein, your body may not have the energy it needs, leading to overall tiredness and weakness.

6. Slow Healing: Protein is necessary for tissue repair. Insufficient protein can slow down wound healing and recovery from injuries.

7. Edema: Protein helps maintain fluid balance in your body. A deficiency can cause swelling, especially in the legs and feet.

8. Mood Changes: Amino acids from protein are precursors to neurotransmitters. A lack of protein can lead to mood swings, anxiety, and depression.

9. Bone Weakness: Protein is important for bone health. Insufficient protein can lead to weaker bones and a higher risk of fractures.

10. Difficulty Losing Weight: Protein boosts metabolism and helps maintain muscle mass during weight loss. Not getting enough protein can make it harder to lose weight and keep it off.

Plant-Based Protein

While animal proteins are complete by nature, there are powerful plant-based foods that provide essential amino acids and support muscle growth, recovery, and overall health. These nutrient-dense options are ideal for anyone looking to boost protein intake through vegetables, herbs, and greens.

1. Beets & Beet Greens – Dietary Nitrates & Antioxidants

Why: Beets are rich in dietary nitrates that convert to nitric oxide during exercise, improving blood flow and performance. Beet greens provide vitamins A and C, supporting immunity and tissue repair.

How: Grate raw beets into salads, blend into smoothies, or pair with chocolate protein powder and berries for a rich, energizing mix.

2. Microgreens & Sprouts – Enzyme-Rich & Anti-Inflammatory

Why: These young greens are packed with enzymes that aid digestion and enhance amino acid absorption. Compounds like sulforaphane offer powerful antioxidant and anti-inflammatory effects.

How: Add sprouts and microgreens to wraps, sandwiches, burgers, or grain bowls.

3. Barley Grass & Wheatgrass – Minerals & Chlorophyll

Why: These grasses are high in antioxidants and minerals such as iron, calcium, and magnesium—key nutrients for muscle function and endurance.

How: Use in smoothies as powdered or juiced forms, or blend with other greens in salad wraps or drinks.

4. Parsley, Chives & Leeks – Lysine for Joint Recovery

Why: These herbs contain lysine, an essential amino acid that supports connective tissue growth and aids joint recovery.

How: Use parsley and chives as fresh garnishes. Add leeks to sautéed vegetable dishes for a mild, sweet flavor.

5. Spirulina – Amino Acids & Metabolic Support

Why: This blue-green algae is rich in protein and contains vitamin B6, which supports metabolism and amino acid utilization.

How: Add spirulina or chlorella powder to smoothies or juices. Rotate them for variety in taste and nutrient profiles.

6. Spinach – Arginine for Growth & Repair

Why: Spinach provides plant-based arginine, an amino acid that promotes growth hormone release and supports protein synthesis.

How: Sauté spinach with cooked grains and legumes. Top with herbs, avocado, or olives for a nutrient-dense meal.

Vegetarian Protein Pairings – Complete Amino Combinations

To build a complete amino acid profile, combine plant proteins strategically:
- Legumes + Whole Grains (e.g., lentils and rice)
- Nuts + Seeds + Leafy Greens
- Hummus + Whole Grain Pita
- Quinoa + Black Beans
- Oats + Chia or Hemp Seeds

Research Linking Plant Protein to Longevity and Healthy Aging

Large-scale studies consistently show that higher intake of plant-based protein—especially when replacing animal protein—is linked to lower mortality, healthier aging, and longer life.

JAMA Internal Medicine (2020, U.S. cohort, 416k adults): Replacing 3% of daily energy from animal with plant protein → **10% lower all-cause mortality, 11–12% lower CVD mortality.**

Nurses' Health Study (AJCN, 2024, 48k women): 3% higher plant protein intake → **38% higher odds of healthy aging**; replacing animal protein improved odds by **22–58%.**

Global Study (Scientific Reports, 2023, 101 countries): Plant protein availability correlated with **longer adult life expectancy**; animal protein linked to shorter adult lifespan despite childhood survival benefits.

Chinese Cohort (Eur J Nutr, 2024): Higher plant protein intake associated with **slower biological aging**; swapping red/processed meat for whole grains/nuts slowed aging markers.

Meta-analysis (Front Nutr, 2022): Replacing 5% of energy from animal with plant protein → **16% lower risk of cognitive decline.**

Harvard/JAMA Meta-analysis (2020): Each 3% increase in plant protein → **5% lower risk of premature death.**

Conclusion: Across populations and study types, greater plant protein intake is consistently associated with reduced mortality, slower biological aging, and better physical and cognitive health. Incorporating legumes, tofu, tempeh, nuts, seeds, and whole grains supports long-term vitality.

Plant Proteins with the Highest Complete Amino Acids

These plant-based protein sources contain all nine essential amino acids in adequate amounts, qualifying them as complete proteins. They are especially valuable in vegetarian and vegan diets for supporting muscle repair, immune function, and overall health.

Top Complete Plant Proteins

1. Quinoa

A rare grain that is a true complete protein. It's high in lysine and methionine, two amino acids often lacking in other plant foods. Also rich in fiber and iron.

2. Soy (Tofu, Tempeh, Edamame)

The most thoroughly researched plant protein. Rich in leucine, essential for muscle growth and repair. Offers high-quality protein comparable to animal sources.

3. Buckwheat

Despite its name, buckwheat is gluten-free and not related to wheat. It contains all essential amino acids, especially lysine, which is limited in most grains.

4. Amaranth

An ancient grain high in methionine and lysine. It provides a complete protein and is easily digestible.

5. Hemp Seeds

A highly digestible protein with all essential amino acids. While slightly lower in lysine, it is rich in healthy fats and ideal for supporting energy and recovery.

6. Chia Seeds

Contains all nine essential amino acids, although the overall protein content per serving is lower. Best used to complement other high-protein sources.

7. Spirulina: A Nutrient-Dense Powerhouse

Spirulina is a blue-green algae packed with complete protein, containing all **nine essential amino acids**. It offers about **60–70% protein by weight**, making it one of the most protein-dense foods on the planet. Unlike many plant-based sources, spirulina also delivers a rich supply of **B vitamins, iron, antioxidants**, and **phycocyanin**, a powerful anti-inflammatory compound. It's easy to digest, supports immune health, boosts energy, and may aid in muscle recovery. Ideal for those seeking a clean, plant-based protein with additional health benefits.

> **Note:** These plant proteins are complete on their own, but many people still benefit from combining complementary sources—like rice and beans—to maximize amino acid balance across the day.

Chapter 17
MEAL REPLACEMENTS

A selection of **nutrient-dense**, versatile foods that align with the **Mediterranean die**t and are **suitable for many other healthy eating styles**. These options support weight management, energy, digestion, and overall wellness.

Animal Protein Sources

Lean & High-Quality:

Poultry
Chicken breast or thigh
Turkey breast
Duck, quail, rabbit (lean cuts, less frequent)
   Fish
Salmon (wild-caught, sockeye, Atlantic)
Tuna (fresh or canned in olive oil)
Sardines
Mackerel
Cod
   Seafood
Shrimp
Scallops
Mussels

Octopus

Squid (calamari)

Eggs & Dairy

Eggs (whole & egg whites)

Greek yogurt (unsweetened, high-protein)

Cottage cheese

Feta cheese

Halloumi cheese

Ricotta cheese

Kefir (unsweetened)

Red Meat

Grass-fed beef (lean cuts: sirloin, flank, top round)

Lamb loin or chops

Pork tenderloin (limited for Mediterranean focus)

Bison, venison (more common in high-protein or Paleo variants)

Plant-Based Proteins

- Chickpeas

- Lentils

- Black beans

- Cannellini beans

- White beans

- Spirulina

- Edamame (more common in vegetarian diets)

- Tofu, Tempeh (not traditionally Mediterranean, but included in plant-based variations)

Carbohydrate Sources

(Whole, Fiber-Rich & Low Glycemic)

Whole Grains & Starches

- Quinoa
- Farro
- Bulgur
- Brown rice
- Wild rice
- Whole grain pasta
- Whole grain pita bread
- Whole wheat bread
- Sourdough bread
- Oats (steel-cut or rolled)
- Sweet potatoes
- Purple potatoes
- Whole corn

Legumes

- Lentils
- Chickpeas

- Black beans
- White beans

Root Vegetables

- Carrots
- Beets
- Parsnips
- Turnips

Squashes

- Butternut squash
- Acorn squash
- Spaghetti squash

Nightshades & Other Veggies

- Bell peppers
- Tomatoes
- Cucumbers
- Zucchini
- Eggplant
- Onions
- Garlic

- Mushrooms

Leafy Greens

- Spinach
- Kale
- Swiss chard
- Arugula

Cruciferous & Fiber-Rich Veggies

- Brussels sprouts
- Broccoli
- Cauliflower
- Cabbage
- Artichokes
- Green beans

Fat Sources

Use these to replace other fats in your diet

- Avocado oil
- Avocados
- Olive oil
- Coconut oil

- MCT oil
- Chia seeds
- Flaxseeds
- Hemp seeds
- Walnuts
- Almonds
- Pecans
- Macadamia nuts
- Brazil nuts
- Pumpkin seeds
- Sunflower seeds
- Natural peanut butter
- Almond butter
- Tahini
- Olives
- Full-fat plain Greek yogurt
- Full-fat cottage cheese
- Whole eggs
- Fatty fish (salmon, sardines, mackerel)
- Grass-fed butter
- Ghee

Food Hacks

- **Portion Control:** Eat smaller portions—even healthy foods can cause weight gain in excess.

- **Eat More Protein:** Include lean meats, fish, eggs, some beans, and legumes to stay full longer.

- **Increase Fiber:** Add vegetables, fruits, whole grains such as sprouted bread, and legumes for fullness and better digestion

- **Limit Processed Foods**: Stick to whole, unprocessed options.

- **Stay Hydrated:** Drink plenty of water.

- **Eat Mindfully**: Savor your meals without distractions to recognize when you're full.

- **Plan Meals:** Prep ahead to avoid unhealthy choices when hungry.

- **Limit Sugary Drinks:** Skip sugary drinks and fruit juices; choose water, herbal tea, or black coffee.

- **Eat More Vegetables:** Nutrient-dense and low in calories.

- **Don't Skip Meals:** Regular, balanced meals prevent overeating later.

- **Watch Liquid Calories:** Choose healthier alternatives to alcohol, specialty coffees, and smoothies.

Over the years, I've developed a handful of simple, sustainable food habits that help me stay consistent. These aren't fancy—they're practical and repeatable. They work for me, and maybe they'll work for you, too. Just remember: it's not about doing what *I* do—it's about what *you* can stick with, medium to long term. Sustainability is the real key.

Simplify Your Proteins: To save time and reduce decision fatigue, I usually eat the same protein throughout the week. Some people need more variety, and that's totally fine. Do what keeps you consistent.

Here's how I prep my proteins:
- **Lean Beef Patties (93% lean / 7% fat):** I season them, form the patties, some go in the fridge, some in the freezer.

- **Chicken Thighs or Breasts:** Same deal—seasoned how I like them; keep raw [cooked to order], or freeze.

I might eat beef on Monday, chicken on Tuesday—it depends on how I feel. The important part is making sure I hit my daily protein goal.

Easy Veggie Dip with Flavor and Fat
Veggies are great—but let's be honest, they're even better with a good dip:
- Start with sour cream—fat-free, 2%, or 5%. I prefer some fat in mine, since healthy fats help your body absorb the nutrients in vegetables. Transfer some sour cream to a separate container and stir in a little from a packet of quality dried French onion soup mix, mix well and let it sit in the fridge for about 48 hours to let the flavors fully develop. **Note:** French onion soup mix is usually high in sodium, so if you're watching your salt intake, this might not be the best option—or look for a low-sodium version. Also try cottage cheese as a base; French onion hummus, and avocado dip. I enjoy them with carrots, raw cauliflower, and broccoli. Just make sure to choose low-sodium versions.

A good trick for bringing food to work is having your salad in Tupperware with the dressing on the bottom or in separate containers. I might put it on the bottom, but I don't shake it until I'm ready to eat. I would also keep foil packets of tuna or salmon in the office, then shake them up for a great meal. I did that three or four times a week for many years. Also, keep protein bars and more at the office, many ideas described below – skip the food machines and eating lunch out all the time. For many years, I have also brought bananas, apples, and natural, organic almond butter. One of my favorites.

> Another thing I've used for decades and still do today is that I *usually don't eat two or three-course meals*, <u>but that's just me</u>, except on holidays. I divide my protein, salad, and carbs into breakfast, lunch, and dinner. So, a

> one-course meal feeds me for the entire day, keeping me from ever having a weight problem. I still get my fruit and Veggies but I spread it all out.

Protein Hacks

Add Egg Whites to Whole Eggs or Oatmeal

Egg whites are nearly pure protein (about 3g per white) with zero fat and minimal calories.

Hack: Add 2–4 egg whites to whole eggs to boost protein without increasing fat. You can also stir them into hot oatmeal while cooking — they blend smoothly and make it creamy without changing flavor.

Why it matters: Great for satiety and muscle support with minimal calories.

Use Greek Yogurt Wisely

Greek yogurt can be a great source of protein (15–20g per serving), but not all brands are created equal.

Hack: Choose plain, unsweetened Greek yogurt and add your own fruit or a dash of cinnamon.

Caution: Many flavored brands are loaded with sugar — check labels for <7g sugar and high protein content.

Add Protein Powder to Regular Foods

Protein powders can easily be added to meals without changing their nature.

Hack: Mix a scoop into:

- Oatmeal

- Coffee (blend or stir with hot milk or water)

- Greek yogurt (for a "pro-yo" snack)

- Pancake or waffle batter

- Homemade granola or nut butter

Bonus: Use unflavored powder for savory foods like soups or mashed potatoes.

Keep Portable Lean Protein Snacks on Hand

Jerky and tuna packets are convenient, but watch sodium levels.

Hack: Choose low-sodium jerky (ideally <300mg per serving) or no-salt-added tuna. Try vacuum-packed grilled chicken strips or hard-boiled eggs.

Why it works: Shelf-stable, high-protein, and convenient for busy days.

Blend Cottage Cheese into Foods: Cottage cheese is high in casein protein and blends easily.

Hack:

- Blend ½ cup into a smoothie for 12–15g protein

- Mix into pancake or muffin batter

- Stir into scrambled eggs or mashed potatoes

Pro Tip: Use low-sodium, 2% cottage cheese for taste and nutrition.

Use High-Protein Wraps or Tortillas

Hack: Swap your regular wrap for a high-protein, low-carb tortilla (e.g., chickpea or flaxseed flour). Some brands offer 10–12g of protein per wrap.

Use it for: Breakfast burritos, quesadillas, or lean meat and veggie wraps.

Bake with Chickpea or Lentil Flour

Hack: Substitute part of your flour with chickpea or lentil flour in baking.

Why it helps: Adds protein and fiber — ¼ cup has about 5–6g protein. Great in pancakes, muffins, fritters, or crepes.

Add Hemp, Chia, or Flaxseeds

Hack: Add 1–2 tablespoons to oatmeal, yogurt, smoothies, or salads.

- **Hemp seeds:** 10g protein per 3 tbsp

- **Chia seeds:** 5g protein + omega-3s

- **Flaxseeds:** 4g protein + fiber and lignans

Note: Blend or soak flax/chia for best digestion.

Use Edamame or Roasted Chickpeas as Snacks

Hack: Keep shelled edamame or roasted chickpeas on hand.

- ½ cup edamame = 9g protein

- 1 oz roasted chickpeas = 6g protein
  Why it works: Crunchy, satisfying, and plant-based.

Replace Croutons with Protein-Rich Toppings

Hack: Instead of croutons, top salads with:

- Roasted tofu cubes

- Grilled chicken strips

- Hard-boiled eggs

- Roasted chickpeas or seeds
  Why it works: Adds crunch and meaningful protein.

Prepare Protein Shakes for the Week

I like adding ground flaxseed or chia seeds, bananas, and/or strawberries. I often buy frozen berries because they're picked at peak ripeness.

How I Make Protein Shakes: I use unsweetened vanilla almond milk and vanilla protein. Since I enjoy vanilla, it's easy to add fruit like 1–2 bananas or frozen berries. I make enough for 1–2 weeks, storing them in screw-top plastic containers and freezing them.

Choose Smart Protein Bars

Hack: Look for bars with 20–30g protein and low single-digit sugar.

Weight to Calorie Burn Reference

Use this quick guide to estimate fat-loss calorie burn:

- 0.5 lb fat = ~250 calories

- 1 lb = ~500 calories

- 1.5 lbs = ~750 calories

- 2 lbs = ~1,000 calories

Simplify Your Proteins:

To reduce decision fatigue, I often eat the same proteins for a week at a time.

How I prep them:

- **Lean beef patties (93/7):** Season, form, and freeze or refrigerate

- **Chicken thighs/breasts:** Season and prep ahead—some frozen, some cooked fresh

I might rotate proteins by day, but the goal is hitting my daily protein target.

My Sweet Tooth Cheats

Frozen Red Grapes for Snacking: I wash red seedless grapes, freeze them in Tupperware, and let them thaw slightly before eating. They're cold, satisfying, and naturally sweet.

Frozen Nectarines or Peaches for Cravings: Peel and slice fruit into thin strips ($\frac{1}{8}$ inch), freeze them flat on a sheet, then transfer to a container.
They may discolor, but the flavor holds. Let one melt slowly in your mouth—it's a sweet, healthy fix.

Low-sugar yogurt with thawed frozen berries. Don't assume all Greek yogurt is healthy—some have more sugar than regular yogurt. Frozen fruit is picked in season, so you get maximum flavor and nutrients. Combined with yogurt, you get probiotics, antioxidants, and a dessert that satisfies almost any sweet craving.

Another is **microwaving (to soften) a good protein bar and topping it with sugar-free ice cream.**

Nutritious Power Bowls & Snacks

These versatile bowls can be adjusted based on your dietary needs and preferences. Just mix and match the ingredients you have on hand to create a balanced meal quickly!

Protein: Grilled chicken or chickpeas

Fat: Olive oil or avocado

Carbohydrates: Quinoa or brown rice

Extras: Cucumber, cherry tomatoes, red onion, feta cheese, olives, and a squeeze of lemon juice

Mexican Fiesta Bowl

Protein: Black beans or grilled shrimp

Fat: Avocado or a dollop of Greek yogurt

Carbohydrates: Brown rice or whole grain tortilla strips

Extras: Corn, diced tomatoes, red bell peppers, shredded lettuce, cilantro, and a squeeze of lime juice

Asian-Inspired Bowl

Protein: Tofu or grilled salmon

Fat: Sesame oil or cashews

Carbohydrates: Brown rice or soba noodles

Extras: Edamame, shredded carrots, cucumber, red cabbage, green onions, and a drizzle of soy sauce or teriyaki sauce

Harvest Bowl

Protein: Grilled chicken or lentils

Fat: Pumpkin seeds or tahini dressing

Carbohydrates: Sweet potato or farro

Extras: Kale, apple slices, dried cranberries, goat cheese, and a sprinkle of cinnamon

Classic Protein Bowl

Protein: Hard-boiled eggs or turkey slices

Fat: Avocado or a drizzle of olive oil

Carbohydrates: Brown rice or whole grain couscous

Extras: Spinach, cherry tomatoes, shredded carrots, cucumber, and a dash of balsamic vinaigrette

Greek Yogurt Bowl (for a sweet option)

Protein: Greek yogurt

Fat: Chopped nuts (almonds, walnuts)

Carbohydrates: Granola or oats

Extras: Fresh berries, honey, chia seeds, and a sprinkle of cinnamon

Vegan Power Bowl

Protein: Tempeh or black beans

Fat: Avocado or hemp seeds

Carbohydrates: Quinoa or barley

Extras: Mixed greens, roasted red peppers, shredded beets, sunflower seeds, and a tahini dressing

Breakfast Power Bowl

Protein: Scrambled eggs or smoked salmon

Fat: Avocado or a sprinkle of chia seeds

Carbohydrates: Sweet potato hash or whole grain toast

Extras: Spinach, cherry tomatoes, green onions, and a squeeze of lemon

How to Eat Out Without Blowing It

Eating out doesn't have to derail your health goals. Use this simple, practical guide to stay on track while still enjoying your meal.

The 5-Step Smart Choice Guide:

Prioritize Protein

Choose grilled, baked, or roasted proteins:

– Chicken, fish, turkey, eggs, lean beef, tofu

– Avoid fried, breaded, or heavily sauced options

Go Green

– Ask for extra vegetables or a side salad

– Swap fries or chips for steamed greens, sliced cucumbers, or a fresh fruit cup

Watch the Sauces

– Ask for sauces and dressings on the side

– Choose olive oil, vinegar, lemon juice, or salsa for flavor

– Skip creamy dressings, cheese sauces, and sugary glazes

Be Smart About Carbs

– Choose whole grains like brown rice or quinoa

– Skip the breadbasket or eat only a small piece

– Avoid sugary drinks; stick with water, tea, or sparkling water

Control Your Portions

– Ask for a to-go box and put half your meal aside before eating

- Consider ordering from the appetizer or small plates menu
- Eat slowly and stop when you feel about 80% full

Quick Swaps to Remember

Instead of fried or heavy meals, make these smart substitutions:

- Fried chicken sandwich → Grilled chicken wrap or bun-less grilled chicken

- Fries → Side salad or roasted vegetables

- Soda → Water with lemon or unsweetened tea

- Pasta Alfredo → Grilled protein with veggies

- Cheeseburger → Lettuce-wrapped burger with avocado and a side salad

Bonus Tips for Eating Out

- Review the menu online before you go to decide in advance

- Don't arrive overly hungry; have a small healthy snack if needed

- Avoid all-you-can-eat buffets or large combo meals

- Focus on your company and conversation—not just the food

- One meal won't make or break your goals; aim for better, not perfect

- It's okay to leave food on your plate.

Enjoy Yourself: Eating out is also about the experience and connection. Focus on your company and the enjoyment of your meal without guilt.

Making thoughtful choices allows you to enjoy dining out while staying aligned with your health and fitness

Chapter 18
SAFE & SUSTAINABLE FAT LOSS

Losing fat isn't just about the scale—it's about protecting your health, preserving strength, and ensuring the results last. According to the **Mayo Clinic**, the safest and most effective rate of fat loss is **1 to 2 pounds per week**, or approximately **4 to 8 pounds per month**. This guideline is backed by decades of clinical research and real-world results.

Why That Range Works:

- A **caloric deficit of 500 to 1,000 calories per day** results in 1 to 2 pounds of fat loss per week.

- This approach protects your **muscle mass**, prevents **nutrient deficiencies**, and supports a **healthy metabolism**.

- Mayo Clinic emphasizes that slower weight loss leads to more sustainable, long-term success and is less likely to result in rebound weight gain.

Why 20–30 Pounds a Month Is Dangerous:

Promises of losing 20 to 30 pounds in just one month may sound appealing—but they are dangerous, misleading, and harmful to your body. Here's why:

- **Muscle Loss** – Rapid weight loss often results in muscle breakdown, which slows metabolism and weakens your body.

- **Gallstones** – Extreme dieting raises the risk of gallstone formation, especially in individuals with obesity.

- **Heart Strain** – Quick weight loss can disrupt electrolytes, strain the heart, and trigger arrhythmias.

- **Fatigue & Brain Fog** – Excessive restriction leads to low energy, irritability, poor focus, and burnout.

- **Rebound Weight Gain** – The faster the loss, the higher the chance of gaining it back—often with additional fat and reduced metabolic rate.

The Mayo Clinic Diet follows two structured phases:

1. **Lose It! Phase** – A two-week kickstart, typically resulting in a modest 6 to 10-pound loss by adopting healthy behaviors.

2. **Live It! Phase** – A long-term program focusing on losing 1 to 2 pounds per week with lasting lifestyle changes.

This method respects your body's biology and avoids the crash-and-burn cycle common with trendy or extreme diets.

> Bottom Line: Losing 20 to 30 pounds in a month is not true fat loss—it's extreme stress on the body. It sacrifices lean muscle, disrupts metabolism, and raises the risk of long-term setbacks. Real, lasting results are built gradually with consistency and discipline. Lasting transformation is earned over time, not forced in a rush.

References

1. Mayo Clinic Staff. *Weight loss: Choosing a diet that's right for you.* Mayo Foundation for Medical Education and Research, 2023.

2. Mayo Clinic Staff. *Gallstones: Causes and complications.* Mayo Foundation for Medical Education and Research, 2023.

3. Mayo Clinic Staff. *Calories and weight loss: How to balance intake and activity.* Mayo Foundation for Medical Education and Research, 2023.

4. Centers for Disease Control and Prevention. *Healthy Weight – Losing Weight*. U.S. Department of Health & Human Services, 2022.

Fat Loss Facts & Spot Reduction Myths

1. **The Myth of Spot Reduction:** People often want to lose fat from specific areas like the stomach, hips, or thighs. However, spot reduction is a myth; regardless of targeted exercises, you cannot control where your body loses fat.

2. **Why Spot Reduction Doesn't Work:** Fat loss occurs systemically, not locally. When your body burns fat, it does so throughout the body, depending on genetics, hormone levels, and overall caloric balance.

For example, doing 1,000 crunches daily won't specifically reduce fat around your stomach. Instead, it will strengthen the muscles underneath, but the fat covering them may remain unless you reduce your overall body fat percentage.

3. **How to Reduce Fat Effectively:** To reduce fat in any area, focus on overall fat loss through:

- Caloric Deficit: Burn more calories than you consume by combining proper nutrition with regular exercise.

- Strength Training: Build muscle across your entire body, which increases your metabolic rate and helps you burn more calories.

- Cardiovascular Exercise: To increase calorie expenditure, engage in activities like walking, running, cycling, or swimming.

4. **Importance of Core Training:** Even though you cannot spot reduce, strengthening your core has significant benefits:

What Is the Core? The muscles of the trunk—primarily the abdominals, obliques, lower back, pelvic floor, diaphragm, and deep stabilizers—that support posture, protect the spine, and transfer force between the upper and lower body.

Training the Core: Core exercises, like planks, deadlifts, or rotational movements, strengthen the area but won't specifically burn belly fat.

5. A Personal Example: Decades ago, I focused on intense abdominal contractions during most exercises for a year, altogether avoiding crunches and any direct ab training. Yet, my abdominal muscles remained firm. This micro self-study may suggest that strengthening the ABS doesn't always require targeted exercises. I engaged my ABS much more than usual during this experiment in virtually every exercise, including punches, kicks, dumbbell chest presses, overhead presses, bicep curls, triceps, etc.. Engaging your ABS also supports core stability without detracting from the specific exercise. To this day, I continue to train myself and clients in this manner. I recommend giving it a try!

Another point I'd like to stress is that your ABS can be firm but not necessarily profoundly defined like a bodybuilder's. If you want your abdominal muscles to show more, you must incorporate a lot of resistance training into your ABS routine. ***Remember, abdominal muscles are not all about high reps; they're about intensity.***

6. Managing Expectations, It's essential to set realistic goals:

- Balanced Fat Loss: You won't achieve a six-pack or slim hips without reducing your overall body fat percentage.

- Genetic Factors: Genetics significantly determines where your body stores and loses fat first.

- Holistic Approach: Focus on full-body strength training, a healthy diet, and regular cardio rather than obsessing over specific areas.

The Takeaway. Nobody achieves a six-pack while still carrying excess fat in other areas like their hips, thighs, or arms. Fat loss is a whole-body process that requires patience, consistency, and a well-rounded approach to diet and exercise.

Remember: The key is overall fat loss through a mix of strength training, cardiovascular exercise, and a balanced diet. Building core strength improves stability, posture, and athletic performance, but it's important to understand that spot reduction isn't possible. A holistic approach will move you closer to your fitness goals. Stay dedicated, stay consistent, and the results will come.

Skipping Morning Carbs for Fat Loss

Strategically timing carbohydrate intake can enhance fat loss and improve workout performance. While total calorie intake and macronutrient balance matter most, carb timing influences how your body burns fat and builds lean muscle.

Why Skip Carbs in the Morning?

Prolongs Fat Burning: After an overnight fast, insulin levels are low. Avoiding carbs at breakfast helps the body stay in a fat-burning state longer.

Enhances Insulin Sensitivity: Delaying carbs until later in the day—especially post-workout—improves blood sugar control and favors glycogen storage over fat storage.

Provides Steady Energy & Reduces Cravings: A protein- and fat-rich breakfast (eggs, avocado, lean meats) stabilizes blood sugar, improves focus, and reduces cravings later in the day.

The Power of Post-Workout Carbohydrates

Replenishes Glycogen Stores

After resistance training or HIIT, your muscles are highly receptive to carbohydrates. This is the ideal time to replenish glycogen stores without promoting fat storage.

Accelerates Recovery

Carbs consumed post-workout help reduce cortisol levels, minimize muscle breakdown, and speed up recovery—especially when paired with a quality protein source.

Supports Muscle Growth and Metabolic Health

The combination of carbs and protein post-workout promotes muscle repair and growth. Over time, this enhances your metabolic rate and overall body composition.

Best Practices for Fat Loss and Performance

- Start your day with a **low-carb, HIGH-PROTEIN breakfast** such as eggs, avocado, or lean meats.

- Eat most of your **carbohydrates after workouts**—good choices include sweet potatoes, rice, oats, and fruit.

- Choose **whole-food carbs** over processed or sugary options.

- Maintain a **slight calorie deficit** to drive sustainable fat loss.

Should You Train Fasted?

Fasted training can increase fat oxidation, particularly for workouts under one hour. For longer sessions or endurance-based workouts, consuming a small pre-workout snack—such as a piece of fruit, a small protein snack, or a mix of easily digestible carbs and a bit of protein—can make a noticeable difference. Though **Fasted training can increase fat burned during exercise, fat loss still depends on total calories consumed versus burned over time."**

Metabolic Shift After Weight Loss

Weight loss can trigger **metabolic adaptation**, where metabolism slows and appetite-regulating hormones shift, leading to a plateau despite calorie restriction. This occurs as the basal metabolic rate (BMR) decreases with weight loss, reducing energy expenditure and stalling progress. **To overcome this, reassess dietary habits, boost physical activity, and incorporate resistance training.**

Key strategies include: Adjust caloric intake to match your current metabolic needs. Generally, most **women should not consume less than 1,200 calories per day, and most men should not consume less than 1,500 calories per day** without medical supervision. Try increasing aerobic exercise to **150–300 minutes per week.** Incorporate daily physical activity. Remember: brisk and interval walking are effective activities for weight loss and belly fat reduction.

In a Nutshell:

- **Portion control:** Correct—excess calories, even from "healthy" foods, can cause weight gain.

- **Protein:** Supported by research; higher protein improves satiety and helps maintain muscle mass.

- **Fiber:** Correct—fiber from vegetables, fruits, whole grains, legumes improves fullness and digestion.

- **Limit processed foods:** Accurate—reduces excess calories, sodium, and added sugars.

- **Hydration:** Correct—often mistaken hunger is thirst.

- **Mindful eating:** Evidence supports slower, distraction-free eating for portion control.

- **Meal planning:** Correct—reduces reliance on impulse, high-calorie foods.

- **Limit sugary drinks:** Accurate—liquid sugar strongly linked with obesity and metabolic issues.

- **Vegetables:** Correct—nutrient-dense, low energy density.

- **Don't skip meals:** Supported—skipping can backfire by increasing hunger and overeating later.

- **Watch liquid calories:** Accurate—alcohol, specialty coffees, smoothies add unnoticed calories.

Sabotaging Fat Loss – Hello Metabolism

- Eating too little

- Doing excessive cardio

- Fat-Burning Supplements — Use with Caution

- Skipping meals

These approaches slow the body's ability to burn calories, making fat loss harder and fat gain easier—especially after even minor setbacks.

Understanding Metabolism: Metabolism is the body's process of converting food into energy. This energy fuels everything—breathing, thinking, digestion, movement, and tissue repair. A healthy metabolism allows the body to burn more calories, even at rest. A slowed metabolism stores more energy as fat, especially when calorie intake is too low or activity is extreme.

Fat Loss vs. Weight Loss: Weight loss is not the goal—**fat loss** is. Losing muscle weakens the body and slows metabolism. Muscle is essential: it improves appearance, supports health, and burns more calories even when inactive. The focus should be on reducing body fat while preserving or increasing lean muscle mass.

The Fat Loss Formula: Fat loss occurs when you burn more calories than you consume. This is called a **caloric deficit**. There are two ways to create it:

1. Increase physical activity

2. Slightly reduce calorie intake

The most effective strategy combines both, but also emphasizes **raising your metabolic rate** so your body naturally burns more calories without overtraining or starving.

How to Support Metabolism and Fat Loss

- **Lift weights to build muscle** – Muscle increases resting calorie burn.

- **Eat adequate protein** – Supports muscle preservation and has a higher thermic effect.

- **Avoid extreme diets** – Severe restrictions cause metabolic slowdown and rebound weight gain.

- **Include cardio, but don't rely on it** – Use it to complement resistance training.

- **Prioritize sleep and manage stress** – Poor recovery raises cortisol, which impairs fat loss.

- **Walk** (Sprint if you can)

Bottom Line: You don't need to starve, skip meals, or live on a treadmill. These behaviors backfire.

Sustainable fat loss is about fueling wisely, building lean muscle, staying active, and creating a small, steady calorie deficit. Focus on **training your body to burn more—not just eating less.**

DAILY REMINDER CHART

- PRAY.

- BOWEL MOVEMENT 1st thing every morning: Make it a routine to have a bowel movement once or twice **each morning**. Why in the morning? This way, you won't feel sluggish throughout the day and won't have to stress about when the urge will strike. Additionally, it will feel more refreshing to accomplish this in the a.m., helping your body eliminate waste effectively.

- Drink a glass of filtered WATER 1st thing EACH MORNING.

- Schedule your workout time for the week.

- Plan your meals *(at the <u>beginning</u> of each week, **meal plan**)*

- Drink 8+ glasses of water.

- Limit refined carbohydrates *(refined & simple sugars)*, often called "added sugars".

- Limit saturated fats.

- Nothing white. And overall, nothing processed.

- Be mindful of fruit consumption:

- Fruit is nutritious but should be consumed in moderation due to its sugar content. One or two servings daily are fine, but too much, especially in smoothies, can raise blood sugar. Whole fruits offer **fiber**, vitamins, and minerals, while juicing removes fiber and increases sugar concentration. For those with metabolic issues, choose whole fruits over juices or smoothies to stabilize blood sugar.

- Limit alcohol consumption.

- Breathe deeply throughout the day.

- **Eat whole foods (to as close to as God made it)**

Beloved, I pray that you may prosper in all things and be in good health, just as your soul prospers. (3 john 1:2)

A TRAINER GUIDED BY GOD'S HEART

By Wally B.

In the gym's bright hum, where iron clinks and clatters,
There stands a master whose strength really counts.
With hands like steel and a heart full of grace,
He lifts more than weights—he lifts every face.

Every morning, his clients arrive, eager to try, and under his watch, they reach for the sky.
With patience and wisdom, he guides each set, no failure too daunting, no limit unmet.

His smile is a beacon, his voice steady and calm, a force of compassion, a soul full of charm.
Through sweat and struggle, he stands as a guide, a pillar of strength with kindness by his side.

Employees genuinely value his leadership style, which balances respectful communication with fairness. He builds a caring connection and can always be counted on in this unpredictable world.

No storm can break him, no challenge too great, for inside his heart beats with unwavering resolve. With every rep and every call, he stands tall, lifting others and standing proud through it all.

In the lively atmosphere of the gym, surrounded by sweat and effort, he feels like both a comforting shelter and a refreshing rain during a storm. He is a master—feisty yet caring—a legendary figure in fitness, with a heart that's deeply connected and warm.

EPILOGUE

The Battle That Challenged Everything

I never thought I'd be writing this part. Life doesn't ease in—it crashes. At 71, I felt unshakable. For my 68th birthday, I knocked out 1,000 pushups in about an hour. It wasn't just a number. It was a testament to years of grit, control, and commitment. I did most everything to fortify myself—but the storm still came.

That's the hard truth I want to leave you with: **sometimes, even when you do all you can, life hits anyway**. But strength isn't just built in the gym—it's tested in the aftermath. My battle didn't end with reps and routines. It deepened. And through that fight, I learned that resilience isn't about avoiding the fall. It's about what you do when you're forced to rise again.

Then the stroke hit. Doctors called it moderately significant. Half my body went silent. I couldn't stand. Couldn't walk. I was locked inside a version of myself I didn't recognize.

I won't pretend to be grateful for the stroke, but I am thankful I was ready. Every early workout, every repetition, every quiet decision showing up for 5 decades had fortified me. That strength didn't stop the storm, but it helped me stand inside of it.

For more than two years, I've experienced the aftermath. My body still doesn't move as it used to. Sometimes, I can't help but ask: Why me? Yet, my faith responds. God sends people, both from my past and present, to my thoughts and my path, reminding me of mental endurance. They remind me: **I'm still here. I'm still rising. I'm still fighting.**

Recovery Without a Roadmap

There's no clear playbook for life after a high-level stroke—no protocol for year two or three, when the rehab team is gone and the battle becomes yours alone. So, I draw my own map. I test and track every movement. I modify routines weekly, reassess what works, and adapt on the fly. Progress is slow, sometimes invisible, **but it is definitely there**.

I record every step of progress. This process, rooted in persistence and creativity, enhances my capacity to assist others in discovering their paths at an even higher level. Recently, I started training a client who suffered a devastating stroke. He can't really speak and remains in a wheelchair after four years at about fifty years old. But the fire in his eyes? Unmistakable. Every flicker of effort from him takes more courage than most people will ever understand. Every session with him deepens my resolve. We fight different battles—but we fight beside each other, united by one truth: **Progress is possible.**

A Guide Forged in Fire

The path we are on serves a greater purpose. Once progress is unmistakable, I hope to write a practical manual forged from hard work, challenges, and real-life experiences, rather than theoretical. This guide won't just be for stroke survivors—it'll be for anyone who's been told they're too old, too broken, or past their prime, because I've heard the word *"impossible."* And I've chosen to defy it.

Fitness isn't just about strength. It's about *resilience*. And faith? That's not just comfort—it's the *rock beneath your feet* when everything else shakes. If life hasn't tested you yet, it will. When that day comes, you'll either fall apart or rise. **So train your body. Sharpen your mind. Anchor your soul. We don't get to choose every storm, but we do choose how we stand in it. And tomorrow? We rise again.**

FINAL THOUGHTS

I work out five days a week, and my routine is always evolving to meet my needs. I combine traditional weightlifting with isometrics, resistance bands, balance work, flexibility techniques, and functional movements—each helping me move better and live stronger. I stay tuned in, listening to my body, and making adjustments—not to be perfect, but to stay healthy and feel my best.

I hope that everything I've shared, experienced, and poured into this book will ignite a spark in someone's heart. My wish is that it reaches those who feel broken, stuck, or forgotten—and encourages them to rise from the ashes. The strength you need isn't somewhere outside; it's already within you, just waiting to be embraced.

I believe that during our time on Earth, we're meant to carry the spirit of lifting each other up. We're here to encourage, to help rebuild what's been broken, and to bring life where there's been silence. If this book accomplishes anything, I hope it inspires someone—not just to grow stronger physically, but to rise up from within.

"These things I have spoken unto you, that in Me ye might have peace. In the world ye shall have tribulation: but be of good cheer; I have overcome the world."—John 16:33 (KJV)

"Finally, my brethren, be strong in the Lord, and in the power of His might ."—Ephesians 6:10 (KJV)

"But they that wait upon the Lord shall renew their strength; they shall mount up with wings as eagles; they shall run, and not be weary; and they shall walk, and not faint."—Isaiah 40:31 (KJV)

These verses are not just promises; they are **battle cries** for anyone who has faced hardship and chosen to rise again.

Let this be your reminder: ***The fight is not over. The best is not behind you. And with God, your strength will rise—even when you fall.***

ABOUT THE AUTHOR

Waldimir "Wally" Baskovich was born in the heart of Chicago, where the grit of the city met the enduring strength of his Serbian and Greek heritage. He was raised on resilience. His father, also named Waldimir, lost his leg at age 11 and went on to become a three-time AAU gold medalist in gymnastics and a two-time U.S. Amputee Golf Champion—the first amputee to win a gymnastics gold medal in the 1940s. For a few key years in Wally's childhood, his father woke him each morning for calisthenics, instilling a discipline that would later become his lifeline.

At age five, Wally's family relocated to the coast of Florida, where life remained challenging—marked by hardship, a near-drowning incident at eight, constant bullying, deep insecurity, and a long battle with social phobia. By his late teens, he'd become entangled in the counterculture movement, chasing peace while wrestling with inner chaos.

Between the ages of 19 and 22, everything changed. Wally rediscovered the strength planted in him as a child. Through martial arts, weightlifting, and a powerful spiritual awakening, he found direction, purpose, and healing. He cut ties with destructive influences and began turning pain into discipline, chaos into clarity—a journey that continues over fifty years later.

Since 1979, Wally has studied nutrition and modeled his training approach after fitness legends. Influenced by Jack LaLanne, Bruce Lee, Arthur Jones of Nautilus, and Charles Atlas's dynamic tension principles, he created a methodology rooted in old-school grit, functional strength, and mind-body integration. He also trained in Shotokan Karate and drew deeply from the lessons passed down by his father.

In his 60s, Wally completed 1,000 push-ups in about an hour and 210 pull-ups in just over 30 minutes—not to chase records, but to stay prepared for life. Those feats weren't about ego—they were a reflection of the mindset he lives by: discipline over excuses, consistency over comfort.

He owns and operates a personal training studio focused on functional fitness, specializing in clients over 50, post-rehab recovery, and neurological conditions. In earlier years, he also coached clients for athletic performance, mud runs, and military physical readiness tests.

Wally doesn't train for applause. He trains for clarity, strength, and purpose—and teaches others to do the same. His greatest victories are reflected in lives rebuilt—people who moved again, believed again, and stood taller because someone refused to let them give up.

This mission—to strengthen the body, sharpen the mind, and steady the soul—is the heartbeat of his work, and he'll continue it for as long as God gives him breath.

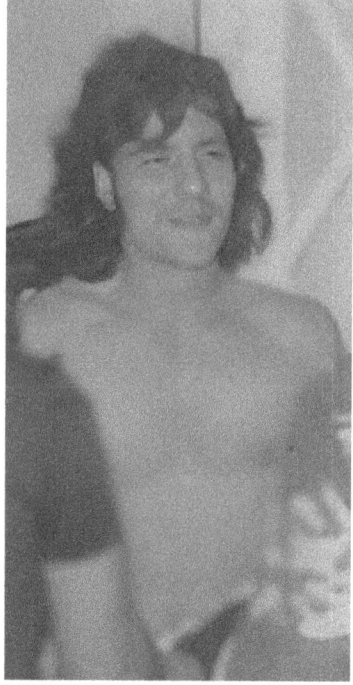

Me as a hippie

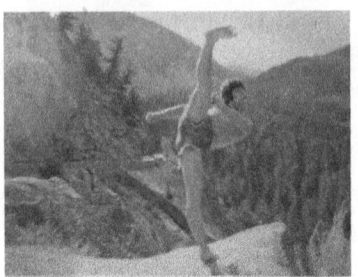

Few years after being a hippie

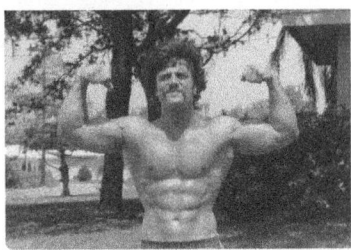

As a bodybuilder

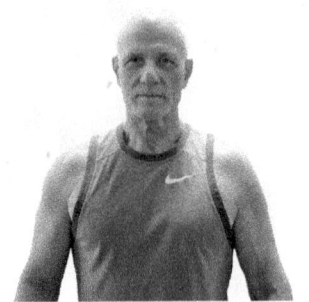

My late sixties

www.ingramcontent.com/pod-product-compliance
Lightning Source LLC
Chambersburg PA
CBHW060947050426
42337CB00052B/1620